THE DIABETES Snack Munch Nibble Nosh Book

RUTH GLICK

Director, Book Publishing, John Fedor; *Associate Director, Consumer Books*, Sherrye Landrum; *Editor*, Laurie Guffey; *Associate Director, Book Production*, Peggy M. Rote; *Composition and Cover Design*, Circle Graphics, Inc.; *Printer*, Transcontinental Printing

Printed in Canada
1 3 5 7 9 10 8 6 4 2

The suggestions and information contained in this publication are generally consistent with the *Clinical Practice Recommendations* and other policies of the American Diabetes Association, but they do not represent the policy or position of the Association or any of its boards or committees. Reasonable steps have been taken to ensure the accuracy of the information presented. However, the American Diabetes Association cannot ensure the safety or efficacy of any product or service described in this publication. Individuals are advised to consult a physician or other appropriate health care professional before undertaking any diet or exercise program or taking any medication referred to in this publication. Professionals must use and apply their own professional judgment, experience, and training and should not rely solely on the information contained in this publication before prescribing any diet, exercise, or medication. The American Diabetes Association—its officers, directors, employees, volunteers, and members—assumes no responsibility or liability for personal or other injury, loss, or damage that may result from the suggestions or information in this publication.

♾ The paper in this publication meets the requirements of the ANSI Standard Z39.48-1992 (permanence of paper).

ADA titles may be purchased for business or promotional use or for special sales. To purchase this book in large quantities, or for custom editions of this book with your logo, contact Lee Romano Sequeira, Special Sales & Promotions, at the address below, or at LRomano@diabetes.org or 703-299-2046.

American Diabetes Association
1701 North Beauregard Street
Alexandria, Virginia 22311

Library of Congress Cataloging-in-Publication Data

Glick, Ruth.
The diabetes snack, munch, nibble nosh book / Ruth Glick.—2nd ed.
p. cm.
ISBN 1-58040-177-5 (pbk. : alk. paper)
1. Diabetes—Diet therapy—Recipes. 2. Snack foods. 3. Appetizers.
4. Desserts. I. American Diabetes Association. II. Title.

RC662.G57 2003
641.5'6314—dc21

2003052125

Contents

Foreword

Snacking is an integral part of the American lifestyle. For people with diabetes, snacking used to be more tightly-controlled, due to fixed insulin regimens and limited oral medication choices. These days, people with diabetes can design more flexible meal plans together with many different insulin regimens and new oral medication choices.

With today's more individualized meal plans, people have a great need for books that provide nutritious, fun, and tasty recipes. *The Diabetes Snack Munch Nibble Nosh Book* provides recipes that are low in fat, calorie-controlled, easy to make, and appetizing to eat. Recipes for people with diabetes can certainly be enjoyed by all, and this book is packed with interesting, flavorful snacks that the whole family can enjoy.

Karmeen Kulkarni, RD, MS, CDE
American Diabetes Association

Preface to the Second Edition

When the American Diabetes Association asked me to revise this book by adding additional snacks, munchies, nibbles, and noshes, I was excited about taking on the project.

I never stop thinking up new ideas for recipes and testing them. Creative cooking is simply a big part of my life. And I particularly like coming up with dishes that can be enjoyed as mini-meals, either on my own or with friends. So I was thrilled by the prospect of having such a wonderful showcase for some of my new creations.

Working on this project was a lot of fun for me. More importantly, since *The Diabetes Snack Munch Nibble Nosh Book* was first published, there has been a shift in thinking about good nutrition. Back when I worked on the first group of recipes, the emphasis in the medical community was on lowering total fat. Now there's more recognition that the type of fat you eat is equally significant.

Limiting saturated fat—from sources such as meat and dairy products—is still important, particularly for people with diabetes. Even more troublesome are the hydrogenated fats (or trans fats) found in many stick margarines and commercial bakery products. But everyone loves sweets. So, as an alternative to store-bought products, I've provided some easy and healthy goodies in this new group of recipes.

At the same time nutritionists were recognizing the health risks of eating trans fats, they were focusing on good fats—fats that can actually help to lower blood cholesterol. These are the polyunsaturated and monounsaturated fats found in oils, such as canola oil and olive oil, and in nuts. Also vital are the omega-3 fatty acids in oily fish such as salmon.

These new guidelines on good and bad fats have influenced my current thinking on what to fix when I want to snack on my own or serve munchies and desserts to my friends. For example, nuts are now an important part of my meal plan since they add both great flavor and great nutrition to many dishes. And I'm always looking for opportunities to serve fish.

Some of my new recipes include a Peanut Butter and Marmalade sandwich, as well as a pie crust made of ground pecans and another crust made of ground almonds. There are also two recipes that use fish: my Mexican Tuna Dip and Salmon Spread.

Another influence on the revision of this book is the glycemic index, which tells you which carbohydrates are absorbed slowly and thus don't cause an immediate need for a large amount of insulin when they are eaten. Since foods like sweet potatoes and beans are low on the glycemic index, I looked for ways to use them—and came up with recipes like my Sweet Potato Pie and my Salsa Bean Dip.

I've made some other nutritional changes since writing *The Diabetes Snack Munch Nibble Nosh Book*. In the first edition, I used no artificial sweeteners. But with this update, I realized I could substantially expand my range of options by using Splenda, a new sweetener that I've found very useful in desserts and other sweets like my Marzipan Candy.

Splenda is made from sugar, although it's very low in carbohydrates and calories. In many recipes, you can use it just the way you'd use sugar, but it does have some limitations. It tends to make cakes rubbery, which is why I haven't included any cakes in this collection. But I've been very pleased with the results in other recipes such as my New York-Style Cheesecake, Sweet Potato Pie, and Cranberry Tart.

And using Splenda, I've been able to make a drink that tastes a lot like mulled cider—only it's not full of sugar because I start with tea, then add spices and a little fruit juice.

You may notice that my recipes that include Splenda use a lot of vanilla extract as well. This is because many people who have tried these dishes say that Splenda can produce an aftertaste, which I've found can be counteracted with vanilla. Note that when I call for Splenda, I use the boxed product, not the packets designed for coffee and tea, since the former replaces an equal amount of sugar. However, this product is very light and tends to fly out of the measuring cup if you're not careful.

As in the first edition of *The Diabetes Snack Munch Nibble Nosh Book*, I've included a wide variety of recipes for you to enjoy. Some are healthier versions of old favorites, like my cheesecakes. Others are dishes I've invented, like my Cranberry Tart and my Tomato Soup with a Difference. The latter is definitely unusual but really good.

All 25 new recipes appear together in the last chapter of this book, called More Scrumptious Snacks. Some are quick snacks, in small portions that you can make and pop into your mouth, like my Peanut Butter and "Marmalade" Sandwich. Other recipes make multiple servings, like my Tuna Dip, Teriyaki Chicken, and Summer Cheesecake. These can be taken to parties, so you'll know there will be something yummy as well as healthy to eat. Or make these dishes and store leftovers in the refrigerator so you can enjoy some now and more later.

I've had a wonderful time working on these recipes. As always, my primary goal has been to create a variety of foods that taste great, because I've followed my old, reliable philosophy that it doesn't matter how good something is for you . . . it has to be yummy if you want people to eat it.

So be my guest, and snack, munch, nibble, and nosh your way through these new recipes—either on your own or with friends.

Acknowledgments

An enormous amount of testing went into the recipes for *The Diabetes Snack Munch Nibble Nosh Book*. I could never have accomplished all the tests and retests without Joe Galitsky, who cooked many of the recipes in my kitchen and offered suggestions for improvements in appearance, taste appeal, and flavor. I also want to thank my friends and family, especially my husband Norman Glick, my friend Binnie Braunstein, and my Thursday Writing Group, who tasted many of these dishes in their various versions and made helpful suggestions and comments.

Introduction

There's a fun side of snacking and a serious part, too. Both get equal time in *The Diabetes Snack Munch Nibble Nosh Book*. If you've got diabetes, snacks may be an essential part of your meal plan. Snacks at mid-morning and in the afternoon help provide energy and prevent low blood glucose. And a little bit of food at bedtime may be important to give the insulin remaining in your body something to work on. What's more, a snack can be vital if you find yourself eating later than your usual mealtime, because a little extra fuel at the right time will keep your blood glucose level from falling too low.

But just like meals, snacks must be carefully considered in the context of your total meal plan. They should be nutritious, and they need to be counted in your daily total of calories, fats, carbohydrates, and proteins, whether you are taking insulin or not.

All of the recipes in *The Diabetes Snack Munch Nibble Nosh Book* follow the guidelines of the American Diabetes Association. Equally important, they're also great-tasting fare you'll want to enjoy often and serve to your friends as well. Included are more than 150 wonderful snacks, appetizers, and even desserts, designed for many different occasions—from a quick afternoon nibble to snacks that will feed a hungry crowd.

You'll find everything from creamy dips and spreads to hearty sandwiches, from chunky salads to tasty snacks. Some will feed the guys on Super Bowl Sunday. Some make great ladies' bridge club treats. Others are after-school specials that are fun for kids to make and eat. In this latter chapter, nutritious foods are presented in fun ways so that youngsters get used to enjoying snacks that are good for them.

All the recipes taste great. And they're an excellent way to increase the variety of beneficial foods in your diet so that your meal plan never becomes boring. Some of the recipes, like Guacamole, Nachos, Stuffed Mushrooms, and Apple Betty, are old favorites presented here in updated versions. Others are intended to expand your tastes and your definition of the snack concept. If you were raised on down-home American food, you may never have thought of fixing a Middle Eastern Sandwich, Eggplant Sticks, or a Quesadilla. Give these recipes a try. They're tasty, satisfying, and a snap to make.

You might also be surprised to find that *The Diabetes Snack Munch Nibble Nosh Book* has a large chapter filled with flavorful salads. But if you've ever grabbed some coleslaw, potato salad, or three-bean salad out of the refrigerator for an afternoon pick-me-up, you'll understand why these dishes make great snacks. You can prepare them ahead and keep them for several days. And they're full of the healthy vegetables you should be eating. What's more, you don't have to worry about dressings that pile on the fat and calories. These salads are different, since they're all healthy but great-tasting alternatives to standard recipes.

One of my goals with *The Diabetes Snack Munch Nibble Nosh Book* was to expand your consumption of vegetables and fruits by including them in a wide variety of recipes throughout the book. In addition, vegetables star in their own chapter. And fruits are featured prominently in many of my baked goods.

Another of my goals was to keep these snacks low in fat. You'll discover I've used a number of simple techniques for doing this. Many recipes call for judicious amounts of reduced-fat and fat-free dairy products, such as Neufchâtel cream cheese, fat-free sour cream, and reduced-fat mayonnaise. Others take advantage of reduced-fat margarine. In many recipes I use tub-style margarine that has 4.5 grams of fat per tablespoon. If you use a brand with a different fat content, the recipes might not work as well due to variations in the water content of the margarine. And tubstyle margarine spreads easier than the stick variety, so you can use less. When I occasionally call for butter, it's always a small amount. But it does make a significant difference in the flavor of the finished product. In recipes calling for mayonnaise, I prefer the reduced-fat variety with 5 grams of fat per tablespoon. Often this mayonnaise is used to add a little bit of fat, and significant flavor, to salads and dips. You could use mayonnaise with less fat, but the results will not be as tasty.

In every case, I've made taste my bottom line. If I tried a recipe with a fat-free product and didn't like it, I retested with a reduced-fat version. And I've been careful to boost flavor with herbs, spices, and other seasonings. Another of my standard techniques is to use a nonstick skillet where pan frying is called for. I test my culinary creations on family, friends, and colleagues and refine recipes according to their comments. Unless a dish has won praise from a broad cross-section of eaters, you won't see it here.

But you'll notice that I haven't tried to remove every smidgen of fat from recipes. You need some fat in your diet, especially monounsaturated fat from olive oil and other vegetable sources. Also, removing all the fat from foods can remove all the taste. It doesn't matter how healthy a recipe is—if it doesn't taste good and no one wants to eat it, you've wasted your time and the ingredients in making it.

In looking through the recipes in *The Diabetes Snack Munch Nibble Nosh Book*, you might be surprised that a number do include sugar and other sweeteners, such as honey or molasses. For many years, sugar was considered the worst possible thing a person with diabetes could eat. More recently, diabetes researchers have taken a closer look at sugar. Sugars, which have a simple molecular structure, are commonly known as simple carbohydrates, while foods such as potatoes, pasta, and bread have complex molecular structures and are called complex carbohydrates or starches. Because of this, it was assumed by doctors that the body must digest and absorb foods with a simple molecular structure faster, thus resulting in a higher blood glucose level, than foods with a complex molecular structure.

However, a panel of experts convened by the American Diabetes Association in 1993 concluded that sugars, when used as part of a regular meal plan and when consumed with other foods, do not harm blood glucose control in people with either type 1 or type 2 diabetes. Sugars are not a special class of food. They are simply a type of carbohydrate. And it is the total amount of carbohydrates eaten that affects blood glucose levels, not where they come from. So it's okay to include some foods with sugar in your meal plan, as long as you work them into your carbohydrate total for the day. That doesn't mean you can have all the sugar you want. But you can substitute sugar for other foods that have approximately the same number of total carbohydrates. If you want to eat a serving of Apple Crisp or Caramel Popcorn, have it instead of a bread roll or a portion of pasta.

You should also be aware that in conventional recipes and store-bought bakery products, sugar is often combined with ingredients that are high in fat, calories, and sodium. But, since both type 1 and type 2 diabetes are risk factors for heart attack and stroke, it's important to limit high-calorie, high-fat foods in your meal plan. In *The Diabetes Snack Munch Nibble Nosh Book* I've cut back on both fat and calories in recipes where I've used sugar. That means you can enjoy treats like Pecan Buns, Peach Cobbler, and Blueberry Muffins that are not only great tasting but also far better nutritionally than traditional versions.

In baked goods made from scratch, like Cranberry-Orange Muffins and Apple Scone Cake, I've increased the fiber by substituting oat bran for some of the white flour. Another strategy I've used is to take advantage of the natural sugars in fruits, which are also high in fiber as well as vitamins and minerals.

Most of my snacks can be eaten as soon as you make them. Many will keep well in the refrigerator for several days. Where applicable, storage directions are always included. Some recipes make only enough for one or two servings but can be easily doubled. Others will feed a crowd.

There are many recipes in *The Diabetes Snack Munch Nibble Nosh Book* that are easy and quick to make. To speed preparation time, I sometimes use the microwave for part of the cooking process, and there's even a chapter of quick, all-microwave recipes. Another tool that's very useful for creating quick snacks is the toaster oven, which I also use in a number of recipes.

Some quick dishes here use convenience foods like prepared pizza sauce, shredded reduced-fat cheese, refrigerator-case biscuits, tortillas, and stuffing mix. I appreciate convenience in the kitchen, and I use these products when I'm in a hurry.

But there's always a nutritional trade-off. And I've come to realize that the dishes I make myself, like Baked Egg Rolls, Turkey Salad, and Shrimp Remoulade, are better for my family than high-fat, high-calorie, high-sugar, high-sodium commercial preparations. Redesigning traditional recipes lets me create healthier but great-tasting versions of old favorites. Look for Better Deviled Eggs, two versions of Guacamole (one with a reduced amount of avocado and one with no avocado at all), Caramel Popcorn, Mustard Pretzels, Tuna Melts, and Pecan Buns.

If you want to know the exact carbohydrate, fat, protein, and sodium content of any recipe, check its nutritional analysis, which was done by a registered dietitian. Note that if I give two alternatives in the ingredients list, such as low-sodium tomato sauce and regular tomato sauce, the analysis is based on the first alternative. And be aware that if you make substitutions, like using reduced-fat milk instead of fat-free milk, the nutrient analysis will be different.

So the next time you have a snack attack, thumb through the pages of this book and pick something you'd like to fix. There are recipes to satisfy every taste and some that will certainly broaden your perception of the munching experience.

Spread It On

Here's a wonderful collection of tasty dips and spreads. All of them make great snacks and will keep in the refrigerator for several days after they're made. Many, like my Guacamole, Lentil Chopped Liver Spread, or Roasted Onion Spread are also perfect for appetizers or buffet parties, where the emphasis is on grazing.

Some recipes are made primarily from high-fiber ingredients like beans and lentils. Others add fiber with celery, green onions, and sun-dried tomatoes. When I use dairy products, it's the fat-free or reduced-fat variety. Each recipe has just enough fat to give it good flavor. For example, I call for reduced-fat sour cream in my Sun-Dried Tomato Paté because it was far less tasty made with the fat-free variety. And my pestos have just enough olive oil to give them a spreadable texture.

In other recipes, I've achieved the flavor I wanted by mixing low-fat products, such as fat-free sour cream and reduced-fat mayonnaise. By the way, I use the type of reduced-calorie mayonnaise with five grams of fat per tablespoon, since I think it tastes close enough to the real thing to produce good results in dips, spreads, and salad dressings.

Preparation Time: 35 minutes

Serves 24

Serving Size: 1 Tbsp

Sour Cream and Roasted Onion Spread

Roasting is a wonderful way to bring out the flavor of foods, like the onions in this simple but delicious spread. Note that the recipe calls for reduced-fat sour cream rather than the fat-free variety I use in most recipes. In this case, the change makes a significant difference in the taste of the spread.

2 cups coarsely chopped onion

1 tsp olive oil

1 cup reduced-fat sour cream

2–3 drops hot pepper sauce

1/4 tsp salt (optional)

1. Preheat the oven to 400 degrees. Spray a shallow 7- by 11-inch baking pan with nonstick spray coating. Add the onions, and toss with oil.
2. Roast the onions, stirring once or twice until they are very soft and beginning to brown, about 35 to 40 minutes. Remove pan from oven, and cool onions slightly.
3. Mix together the sour cream, hot pepper sauce, and salt, if desired. Stir in the onions. Serve warm or chilled on fat-free whole-wheat crackers or toasted French bread slices.
4. Cover and refrigerate leftover spread. Leftover spread will keep in the refrigerator 3 to 4 days. After refrigeration, stir before serving.

Exchanges

Free

Calories 17

Total Fat 1 g

Saturated Fat 0 g

Calories from Fat 9

Cholesterol 3 mg

Sodium 5 mg

Carbohydrate 2 g

Dietary Fiber 0 g

Sugars 1 g

Protein 0 g

Sun-Dried Tomato Paté

Preparation Time: 15 minutes

Serves 8

Serving Size: 2 Tbsp

This spread tastes great on half a bagel, wheat crackers, or as a stuffing for celery or Belgian endive.

1/2 cup dry-packed sun-dried tomatoes

1/4 cup water

1/2 cup reduced-fat sour cream

3 Tbsp reduced-fat mayonnaise

2 Tbsp grated Parmesan cheese

1/2 tsp basil

1 small garlic clove, chopped

1/4 cup finely chopped celery

2 Tbsp chopped chives or sliced green onion tops

1. In a 2-cup measure or similar small microwave-safe bowl, combine the tomatoes and water. Cover with wax paper and microwave on high power 3 to 4 minutes, or until the tomatoes are softened and most of water has been absorbed. Set aside to cool for about 10 minutes.
2. Transfer to a food processor bowl, and process with on-and-off bursts until the tomatoes are chopped. Transfer to a small bowl, and stir in the sour cream, mayonnaise, cheese, basil, and garlic. Stir to mix well. Stir in the celery and chives. Mix well.
3. Serve at once, or cover and refrigerate. Leftover spread will keep in the refrigerator 3 to 4 days.

Exchanges

1 Fat

Calories 50

Total Fat 3 g

Saturated Fat 1 g

Calories from Fat 30

Cholesterol 8 mg

Sodium 138 mg

Carbohydrate 4 g

Dietary Fiber 1 g

Sugars 1 g

Protein 1 g

Preparation Time: 12 minutes

Serves 16

Serving Size: 2 Tbsp

Artichoke and Shrimp Spread

Elegant but easy, this chunky dip can be served on toasted Italian bread slices or fat-free crackers.

1 13- to 14-oz can water-packed artichoke hearts, well drained

1 cup cooked small shrimp

1/4 cup fat-free sour cream

3 Tbsp reduced-fat mayonnaise

1 1/2 tsp Italian seasoning

1 garlic clove, minced

1 tsp instant minced onions

1 tsp balsamic vinegar

1/8 tsp salt, or to taste (optional)

1/8 tsp white pepper

1. Remove and discard the coarse outer leaves from the artichoke hearts. Chop the hearts slightly, and set them aside in a medium bowl. Chop the shrimp slightly, and set them aside with the artichoke hearts.
2. In a small bowl, stir together the sour cream and mayonnaise. Add the Italian seasoning, garlic, onions, vinegar, salt (if desired), and pepper. Stir to mix well. Stir the mixture into the shrimp and artichokes.
3. Cover and refrigerate at least 1/2 hour and up to 12 hours to allow the flavors to blend.
4. Serve on fat-free crackers or toasted Italian bread slices. Leftover spread will keep in the refrigerator 1 to 2 days.

Exchanges

1/2 Polyunsaturated Fat

Calories 26

Total Fat 1 g

Saturated Fat 0 g

Calories from Fat 9

Cholesterol 17 mg

Sodium 86 mg

Carbohydrate 2 g

Dietary Fiber 0 g

Sugars 1 g

Protein 2 g

Cottage Cheese with Dill and Onion

Preparation Time: 12 minutes

Serves 8

Serving Size: 2 Tbsp

Use this flavored cottage cheese to stuff Belgian endive, celery, or the Dugout Canoes on p. 139. For a quicker but slightly less sophisticated version of the dip, you can omit the food processor step and simply mix the ingredients together in a small bowl.

1 cup low-fat cottage cheese

1 Tbsp reduced-fat mayonnaise

2 Tbsp thinly sliced green onion tops

1/2 tsp fresh dill leaves or 1/4 tsp dried dill weed

1/8 tsp ground celery seed

Pinch of salt, or to taste (optional)

2 drops hot pepper sauce (optional)

1. Combine the cottage cheese and mayonnaise in a food processor bowl fitted with a steel blade. Process until almost smooth.
2. Turn mixture out into a small bowl. Add the onion, dill, celery seed, salt (if desired), and hot pepper sauce (if desired). Stir to mix well.
3. Serve at once or cover and refrigerate. The dip keeps up to 3 days in the refrigerator. Stir before serving.

Exchanges

1 Very Lean Meat

Calories 32

Total Fat 1 g

Saturated Fat 1 g

Calories from Fat 10

Cholesterol 3 mg

Sodium 125 mg

Carbohydrate 1 g

Dietary Fiber 0 g

Sugars 1 g

Protein 4 g

Preparation Time:
7 minutes

Serves 8

Serving Size:
1/4 cup

Nacho Dip

Here's a nacho dip that's low in fat and high in flavor. Enjoy it as a snack or serve it as an appetizer.

1 Tbsp cornstarch

1/2 tsp chili powder

1/4 tsp dry mustard

1 cup low-fat (1%) milk

1 1/2 cups shredded reduced-fat sharp Cheddar cheese

2/3 cup mild salsa

2 Tbsp thinly sliced green onion tops

32 large fat-free tortilla chips

1. In a 4-cup measure or similar microwave-safe bowl, stir together the cornstarch, chili powder, and mustard. Add the milk, stirring with a small wire whisk or fork until the corn starch is completely incorporated.
2. Cover with wax paper, and microwave on high power 2 minutes or until the mixture is very hot. Whisk with a small wire whisk. Cover and microwave again for 30 seconds on high power. Whisk. If the mixture has not thickened, repeat heating and whisking process.
3. Add the cheese, and stir until partially melted. Transfer the mixture to a food processor or blender, and process or blend on medium speed until completely smooth. Stir in the salsa and green onion.

Exchanges

1/2 Starch

1 Medium-Fat Meat

Calories 109

Total Fat 5 g

Saturated Fat 3 g

Calories from Fat 46

Cholesterol 16 mg

Sodium 272 mg

Carbohydrate 8 g

Dietary Fiber 1 g

Sugars 2 g

Protein 9 g

4. Transfer the cheese mixture to a glass bowl. Serve warm, or cover and refrigerate 1 to 2 days until needed. To rewarm, cover with wax paper and microwave 1 1/2 to 2 minutes on full power. Stir.
5. To serve as a snack, lay 4 large tortilla chips on a small plate. Pour the cheese sauce over the chips. For an appetizer, guests can dip chips into the warm cheese mixture. If the mixture begins to cool, cover with wax paper, and microwave 30 to 40 seconds. Or keep warm on a warming tray.

Thousand Island Dressing

Preparation Time: 6 minutes

Serves 10

Serving Size: 1 Tbsp

This tangy dressing is not only a snap to make, it's also quite versatile. Use it for dipping fresh vegetables or shrimp, or as a classic salad dressing. The small amount of reduced-fat mayonnaise adds to the richness of the taste. But, if you like, you can make a completely fat-free version without the mayonnaise.

1/2 cup catsup
1/4 cup fat-free sour cream
1 Tbsp reduced-fat mayonnaise
1/2 Tbsp balsamic vinegar
1 small garlic clove, minced (optional)

1. In a small bowl, combine all the ingredients (including the garlic, if desired), and whisk together well to prevent lumps.
2. Refrigerate dressing for up to a week. After refrigeration, stir before using.

Exchanges

1 Vegetable

Calories 23
Total Fat 1 g
Saturated Fat 0 g
Calories from Fat 5
Cholesterol 1 mg
Sodium 163 mg
Carbohydrate 4 g
Dietary Fiber 0 g
Sugars 2 g
Protein 1 g

Guacamole

Preparation Time: 15 minutes

Serves 14

Serving Size: 2 Tbsp

If you love guacamole but hate the accompanying fat and calories, try this alternative that substitutes green peas for most of the avocado. You'll be surprised at how close this recipe comes to the taste and texture of the original.

- 1 1/2 cups frozen peas
- 1 small ripe avocado, peeled, seeded, and cut into chunks
- 1 Tbsp reduced-fat mayonnaise
- 2 tsp lemon juice
- 1/2 tsp cumin
- 1/2 tsp chili powder
- 1 garlic clove, minced
- 1/2 cup mild or medium low-sodium or regular salsa

1. In a small saucepan, combine the peas and 1/4 cup boiling water. Cover, bring to a boil, and simmer 2 minutes. Cool in a colander under cold running water. Drain well.
2. In a food processor container, combine the peas, avocado, mayonnaise, lemon juice, cumin, chili powder, and garlic. Process until blended but not absolutely smooth, stopping and scraping the container sides, if necessary. Stir in the salsa.
3. Cover and refrigerate 1 to 2 hours or up to 24 hours to allow the flavors to blend. The dip will keep in the refrigerator 1 to 2 days. Serve with fat-free tortilla chips.

Exchanges

1/2 Starch

Calories 36
Total Fat 2 g
Saturated Fat 0 g
Calories from Fat 17
Cholesterol 42 mg
Sodium 42 mg
Carbohydrate 4 g
Dietary Fiber 2 g
Sugars 2 g
Protein 1 g

Preparation Time: 5 minutes

Serves 12

Serving Size: 2 Tbsp

Don't Tell 'Em It's Not Guacamole

Here's a surprisingly tasty version of guacamole made with absolutely no avocado at all.

2 cups frozen peas

3 Tbsp reduced-fat mayonnaise

2 tsp lemon juice

1 tsp cumin

1/2 tsp chili powder

1 garlic clove, minced

1/2 cup mild or medium low-sodium or regular salsa

1/4 tsp salt, or to taste (optional)

1. In a small saucepan, combine the peas and 1/4 cup boiling water. Cover, bring to a boil, and simmer 2 minutes. Cool in a colander under cold running water. Drain well.
2. In a food processor container, combine the peas, mayonnaise, lemon juice, cumin, chili powder, and garlic. Process until blended but not absolutely smooth, stopping and scraping the container sides, if necessary. Stir in the salsa and salt (if desired).
3. Cover and refrigerate 1 to 2 hours or up to 24 hours to allow flavors to blend. The mixture will keep in the refrigerator 4 to 5 days. Serve with fat-free corn chips.

Exchanges

1/2 Starch

Calories 37

Total Fat 1 g

Saturated Fat 0 g

Calories from Fat 11

Cholesterol 2 mg

Sodium 68 mg

Carbohydrate 5 g

Dietary Fiber 2 g

Sugars 2 g

Protein 2 g

Salmon Salad

Serve this quick, tasty salad on fat-free whole-wheat crackers, on a half a bagel, or on half of a whole-wheat English muffin. If you like, top with a ripe tomato slice. Or serve on a plate with lettuce, tomato, cucumbers, and any other raw vegetables you like.

1 6-oz can skinless, boneless pink salmon, well drained

1 1/2 Tbsp reduced-fat mayonnaise

1 tsp prepared white horseradish

1 large celery stalk, chopped

2 Tbsp chopped red or other sweet onion

1. Place the salmon in a small bowl. Flake to separate. Add the mayonnaise and horseradish and stir to mix well.
2. Stir in the celery and onion. Serve at once, or cover and refrigerate. Salad will keep in the refrigerator 1 to 2 days.

Preparation Time: 6 minutes

Serves 5

Serving Size: 1/4 cup

Exchanges

1 Lean Meat

Calories 56

Total Fat 3 g

Saturated Fat 0 g

Calories from Fat 27

Cholesterol 17 mg

Sodium 190 mg

Carbohydrate 1 g

Dietary Fiber 0 g

Sugars 1 g

Protein 6 g

Preparation Time: 6 minutes

Serves 3

Serving Size: 2 Tbsp

Exchanges

1 Lean Meat

Calories 48

Total Fat 2 g

Saturated Fat 0 g

Calories from Fat 16

Cholesterol 9 mg

Sodium 117 mg

Carbohydrate 1 g

Dietary Fiber 0 g

Sugars 0 g

Protein 7 g

Tuna Salad

You can serve this tasty tuna salad in a number of different ways. Spread it on a bagel half, mound it on a plate and surround it with lettuce and other vegetables, or use it to make the tuna melts on page 33.

1 3-oz can water-packed tuna, well drained

1 Tbsp reduced-fat mayonnaise

1 Tbsp chopped red bell pepper

1/2 tsp balsamic vinegar

1 Tbsp chopped chives or sliced green onion tops or red onion

1. In a small bowl, flake the tuna with a fork. Combine with the mayonnaise, pepper, vinegar, and chives. Stir to mix well.
2. Serve as an open-faced sandwich or as a salad surrounded by raw vegetables.

Hummus with Roasted Red Peppers

Preparation Time: 10 minutes

Serves 12

Serving Size: 2 Tbsp

Hummus is a Middle Eastern dip that is often made from ground chickpeas (garbanzo beans) and tahini (sesame butter). I prefer the milder flavor of ground sesame seeds. Roasted red peppers make a nice addition to the basic dip.

1 15-oz can chickpeas, washed and drained
1 garlic clove, minced
2 Tbsp olive oil
2 Tbsp water
1 Tbsp lemon juice
1/2 Tbsp sesame seeds
Scant 1/4 tsp salt (optional)
1/8 tsp black pepper
1/4 cup finely chopped roasted red peppers
2 Tbsp finely chopped fresh parsley

1. In a food processor container, combine the chickpeas, garlic, oil, water, lemon juice, sesame seeds, salt (if desired), and black pepper. Process until smooth. Transfer to a medium bowl.
2. Stir in the roasted peppers and parsley. If the spread seems stiff, add a bit more water. Serve at once or cover and refrigerate 2 to 3 hours or up to 24 hours before serving. The spread will keep in the refrigerator for 4 to 5 days. Serve with whole-wheat pita wedges or fat-free crackers.

Exchanges

1/2 Starch

Calories 50
Total Fat 2 g
Saturated Fat 0 g
Calories from Fat 14
Cholesterol 0 mg
Sodium 36 mg
Carbohydrate 7 g
Dietary Fiber 2 g
Sugars 1 g
Protein 2 g

Preparation Time:
16 minutes

Serves 16

Serving Size:
2 Tbsp

Chickpea and Sun-Dried Tomato Spread

This easy spread features the wonderful combination of chickpeas (garbanzo beans) and sun-dried tomatoes. The spread can be served on fat-free crackers, whole-wheat English muffins, or pita bread wedges.

1/3 cup dry-packed sun-dried tomatoes

1 15 1/2-oz can chickpeas, rinsed and well-drained

1 8-oz can low-sodium tomato sauce or regular tomato sauce

2 Tbsp chopped chives

2 tsp olive oil

1/2 tsp Italian seasoning

1/8 tsp salt, or to taste (optional)

2–3 drops hot pepper sauce (optional)

1. In a small microwave-safe bowl, combine the sun-dried tomatoes and 3 Tbsp of water. Cover with wax paper and microwave on high power 1 to 1 1/2 minutes to soften tomatoes slightly. Drain in a colander. When the tomatoes are cool enough to handle, cut them into quarters. Set aside.
2. In a medium bowl or casserole, mash the chickpeas with a fork or potato masher until coarsely mashed. Stir in the reserved sun-dried tomatoes, tomato sauce, chives, oil, Italian seasoning, salt (if desired), and hot pepper sauce (if desired).
3. Serve at room temperature, or cover and refrigerate. Spread will keep in the refrigerator 3 to 4 days. Stir before serving.

Exchanges

1/2 Starch

Calories 42

Total Fat 1 g

Saturated Fat 0 g

Calories from Fat 10

Cholesterol 0 mg

Sodium 52 mg

Carbohydrate 7 g

Dietary Fiber 2 g

Sugars 1 g

Protein 2 g

Lentil Chopped Liver Spread

Although this spread is made of lentils, it tastes remarkably like chopped liver.

1 1/2 cups dried brown lentils, washed and picked over

2 Tbsp instant minced onions

1 garlic clove, minced

1/3 cup liquid egg substitute

3 Tbsp reduced-fat mayonnaise

1/2 teaspoon salt, or to taste (optional)

Dash of pepper, or to taste

1. In a large saucepan, combine the lentils, onions, and garlic. Cover with 4 to 5 cups of water. Bring to a boil. Cover, reduce the heat, and simmer 25 to 30 minutes or until lentils are tender but not mushy. Drain lentils in a colander.
2. Meanwhile, cook the egg substitute in a small nonstick skillet as if making scrambled eggs, breaking the eggs into small pieces.
3. Combine lentils and egg substitute in a medium bowl. Add the mayonnaise, salt (if desired), and pepper. Stir to mix well. Serve at once, or refrigerate several hours before serving.
4. Serve on crackers or bagel halves. The spread will keep in the refrigerator for 3 to 4 days.

Preparation Time: 10 minutes

Serves 32

Serving Size: 2 Tbsp

Exchanges

1/2 Starch

Calories 37

Total Fat 1 g

Saturated Fat 0 g

Calories from Fat 5

Cholesterol 1 mg

Sodium 14 mg

Carbohydrate 5 g

Dietary Fiber 3 g

Sugars 1 g

Protein 3 g

Preparation Time: 16 minutes

Serves 32

Serving Size: 2 Tbsp

Herbed Lentil Spread

Lentils make delicious spreads. The only drawback is their dark brown color. If you like, garnish with chopped parsley or pimentos. This spread goes well with fat-free whole-wheat crackers. It's also wonderful on bagels or rolls.

1/2 lb brown lentils, washed and sorted
1 small onion, chopped
1 garlic clove, minced
2 Tbsp olive oil
1 1/2 Tbsp Worcestershire sauce
1 Tbsp balsamic vinegar
1 tsp Dijon-style mustard
1/4 tsp dried thyme leaves
1/4 tsp dried marjoram leaves
Generous 1/2 tsp salt, or to taste (optional)
1/8 tsp black pepper
2 celery stalks, minced

1. In a large pot, bring 5 cups of water to a boil. Add the lentils, onion, and garlic. Reduce the heat, cover, and simmer lentils 35 to 45 minutes, stirring occasionally, until the lentils are very tender but not mushy. Drain in a colander.
2. Meanwhile, in a medium bowl, stir together the oil, Worcestershire sauce, vinegar, mustard, thyme, marjoram, salt (if desired), and pepper. Stir in the celery and then stir in the lentil mixture. Cover and refrigerate 2 to 3 hours or up to 24 hours before serving. Spread will keep covered in the refrigerator for 4 to 5 days.

Exchanges

1/2 Starch

Calories 33
Total Fat 1 g
Saturated Fat 0 g
Calories from Fat 8
Cholesterol 0 mg
Sodium 11 mg
Carbohydrate 4 g
Dietary Fiber 2 g
Sugars 1 g
Protein 2 g

Tomato and Olive Tapenade

Preparation Time: 12 minutes

Serves 22

Serving Size: 2 Tbsp

I've called for plum tomatoes in this easy, flavorful spread. However, when vine-ripened tomatoes are available in summer, feel free to use them.

5 plum tomatoes, chopped

12 large ripe pitted olives, chopped

2 Tbsp thinly sliced green onion tops

1 small garlic clove, chopped

1 tsp olive oil

2 tsp balsamic vinegar

1/4 tsp salt (optional)

1/8 tsp black pepper

1. In a medium bowl, combine the tomatoes, olives, onion, and garlic. Stir in the oil, vinegar, salt (if desired), and pepper. Transfer to a food processor container, and process with 4 to 5 on-and-off bursts to further blend the vegetables. Do not overblend.
2. Serve immediately on a small slice of toasted Italian bread or whole-wheat crackers. Or cover and refrigerate several hours, then stir before serving. Leftovers will keep in the refrigerator 2 to 3 days.

Exchanges

Free

Calories 9

Total Fat 1 g

Saturated Fat 0 g

Calories from Fat 5

Cholesterol 0 mg

Sodium 23 mg

Carbohydrate 1 g

Dietary Fiber 0 g

Sugars 1 g

Protein 0 g

Preparation Time: 12 minutes

Serves 7

Serving Size: 3 Tbsp

Roasted Summer Vegetable Spread

Roasting works a magical transformation on this chunky vegetable medley. Serve warm on small slices of Italian bread or crackers. Starting the vegetables in the microwave shortens the cooking time. However, if you like, you can omit this step and roast the vegetables for about 40 to 45 minutes.

4 plum tomatoes, chopped

1/2 cup diced zucchini

1/2 cup very thinly sliced onion

1/2 sweet red pepper, chopped

2 tsp olive oil

1/4 tsp dried thyme leaves

1/4 tsp salt (optional)

1/8 tsp black pepper

1. Preheat the oven to 400 degrees. Spray a 7- by 11-inch baking pan with nonstick spray coating and set aside. In a medium bowl, combine the tomatoes, zucchini, onion, pepper, olive oil, thyme, salt (if desired), and black pepper. Toss to mix. Cover with wax paper and microwave 4 to 5 minutes.
2. Transfer the vegetables to the baking pan, and bake for 25 to 30 minutes, stirring occasionally, or until the onion is tender.
3. Serve at once on toasted Italian bread slices or whole-wheat crackers.

Exchanges

1 Vegetable

Calories 33

Total Fat 1 g

Saturated Fat 0 g

Calories from Fat 13

Cholesterol 0 mg

Sodium 5 mg

Carbohydrate 5 g

Dietary Fiber 1 g

Sugars 3 g

Protein 1 g

Mixed Herb Pesto

Preparation Time:
18 minutes

Serves 12

Serving Size:
1 Tbsp

If you've enjoyed pesto in Italian restaurants, you may be surprised by how easy it is to make at home. This recipe is not only flavorful, it's also lower in fat than traditional versions.

2 Tbsp pine nuts

3 garlic cloves

1 1/4 cups packed fresh basil leaves

1/4 cup packed chopped fresh chives or green onions

1/4 cup packed fresh parsley leaves

3 Tbsp freshly grated Parmesan cheese

1 Tbsp fresh lemon juice

Generous 1/4 teaspoon salt, or more to taste

3 Tbsp extra virgin olive oil

1. Spread the pine nuts in a small, nonstick skillet. Cook over medium-high heat, stirring constantly, until the nuts begin to turn brown and smell toasted, about 3 to 4 minutes. Immediately transfer to a plate and cool slightly.
2. Combine the nuts, garlic, basil, chives, parsley, cheese, lemon juice, and salt in a food processor. Process until finely minced. With the processor on, slowly pour the oil through food tube; process until well blended, stopping and scraping down the sides of the container once or twice.
3. Transfer to a small bowl. Serve at room temperature, or cover with a tight seal and refrigerate. Pesto will keep in the refrigerator for 2 to 3 days.

Exchanges

1 Monounsaturated Fat

Calories 49

Total Fat 5 g

Saturated Fat 1 g

Calories from Fat 42

Cholesterol 1 mg

Sodium 73 mg

Carbohydrate 1 g

Dietary Fiber 0 g

Sugars 1 g

Protein 1 g

Preparation Time: 18 minutes

Serves 18

Serving Size: 1 Tbsp

Sun-Dried Tomato Pesto

Sun-dried tomatoes give this easy pesto a distinctive tang. Serve it on crostini (toasted Italian bread slices) or fat-free crackers.

1 cup dry-packed sun-dried tomatoes
1/4 cup water
1 cup packed fresh basil leaves
1/3 cup chopped chives
1/4 cup fat-free Parmesan cheese topping
3 Tbsp extra virgin olive oil
2 garlic cloves, minced
1/8 tsp black pepper

1. In a 2-cup measure or similar small microwave-safe bowl, combine the sun-dried tomatoes and water. Cover with wax paper and microwave on high power 2 minutes or until the tomatoes are slightly softened.
2. In a food processor bowl, process the tomatoes and water until the tomatoes are coarsely chopped. Remove to a small bowl and set aside. In the food processor bowl, combine the basil, chives, Parmesan cheese, oil, garlic, and pepper. Process until chopped.
3. Stir the basil mixture into the tomatoes. Serve at room temperature, or cover and refrigerate until serving. The pesto will keep for 2 to 3 days in the refrigerator.

Exchanges

1/2 Monounsaturated Fat

Calories 36
Total Fat 2 g
Saturated Fat 1 g
Calories from Fat 21
Cholesterol 0 mg
Sodium 87 mg
Carbohydrate 3 g
Dietary Fiber 0 g
Sugars 1 g
Protein 1 g

Sandwich Board

The recipes in this chapter are for sandwiches you can make quickly and eat at once. Most make one or two servings, although a few are designed to feed a crowd. Many, like my Grilled Portobello Mushroom Sandwich and Falafel, are designed to expand your concept of a sandwich.

Some are presented open-faced on a slice of whole-wheat bread. Others are made on half an English muffin, stuffed into a pita pocket, or rolled in a tortilla. If you like, double the recipe and make it for lunch instead of a snack. Or try the Egg 'N Muffin recipes for breakfast.

When possible, make your sandwiches with whole-wheat, mixed grain, or oat bran bread rather than plain white or wheat bread, since this is an easy way to add fiber to your diet.

Preparation Time:
6 minutes

Serves 2

Serving Size:
1 muffin half

Egg 'N Muffin

This spicy egg and muffin sandwich is great for breakfast, lunch, or a snack any time. For crunch, you can also add a little chopped celery to the egg substitute before cooking.

1/2 cup frozen mixed pepper and onion stir-fry

1/3 cup liquid egg substitute

Pinch dry mustard

Pinch black pepper

1 Tbsp catsup

1 whole-wheat or oat bran English muffin, split in half

2 Tbsp reduced-fat shredded Cheddar cheese

1. In a medium nonstick skillet coated with nonstick spray, cook the pepper and onion mixture over medium-high heat until the onion is tender, 2 or 3 minutes.
2. Lower the heat to medium. Add the egg substitute and mustard and cook, stirring occasionally, until the egg is cooked through, about 2 minutes. Remove from heat and stir in catsup.
3. Spread the mixture evenly on open, untoasted English muffin halves. Sprinkle with cheese. Toast in toaster oven or under broiler until cheese is just melted and muffins are warmed.

Exchanges

1 Starch

1 Very Lean Meat

Calories 123

Total Fat 2 g

Saturated Fat 1 g

Calories from Fat 21

Cholesterol 5 mg

Sodium 333 mg

Carbohydrate 17 g

Dietary Fiber 2 g

Sugars 5 g

Protein 10 g

Egg 'N Muffin, Mexican Style

Here's a spicy variation of my basic Egg 'N Muffin sandwich.

Preparation Time: 6 minutes

Serves 2

Serving Size: 1 muffin half

1/3 cup liquid egg substitute

1/4 tsp chili powder

1/8 tsp salt (optional)

3 Tbsp mild or medium salsa

1 whole-wheat English muffin, split in half

2 Tbsp reduced-fat shredded Cheddar or jack cheese

1. In a medium-sized nonstick skillet coated with nonstick spray, stir together the egg substitute, chili powder, and salt (if desired). Cook over medium heat, stirring occasionally, until cooked through, about 2 minutes. Remove from heat and stir in salsa.
2. Spread the mixture evenly on open, untoasted English muffin halves. Sprinkle with cheese. Toast in toaster oven or under broiler until cheese is just melted and muffins are warmed.

Exchanges

1 Starch

1 Very Lean Meat

Calories 115

Total Fat 2 g

Saturated Fat 1 g

Calories from Fat 21

Cholesterol 5 mg

Sodium 307 mg

Carbohydrate 15 g

Dietary Fiber 2 g

Sugars 3 g

Protein 10 g

Preparation Time: 3 minutes

Serves 2

Serving Size: 1 muffin half

Egg 'N Muffin, Italian Style

Here's an Italian-style variation of my basic Egg 'N Muffin sandwich.

1/3 cup liquid egg substitute

1 Tbsp thinly sliced green onion tops

1/4 tsp Italian seasoning

1 whole-wheat English muffin, split in half

1 Tbsp grated Parmesan cheese

2 thin slices fresh tomato

Chopped parsley for garnish (optional)

1. In a medium-sized nonstick skillet coated with nonstick spray coating, stir together the egg substitute, green onion, and Italian seasoning. Cook over medium heat, stirring occasionally, until cooked through, about 2 minutes.
2. Remove from heat, and spread the mixture evenly on open, untoasted English muffin halves. Sprinkle with cheese and top with tomato.
3. Toast in toaster oven or under the broiler until the cheese is just melted and muffins are warmed. If desired, sprinkle with chopped parsley.

Exchanges

1 Starch

1 Very Lean Meat

Calories 106

Total Fat 2 g

Saturated Fat 1 g

Calories from Fat 17

Cholesterol 4 mg

Sodium 248 mg

Carbohydrate 15 g

Dietary Fiber 2 g

Sugars 3 g

Protein 9 g

Grilled Portobello Mushroom Sandwich

Try this extremely versatile recipe for a grilled portobello mushroom sandwich. You can garnish your sandwich with a little balsamic vinegar, Dijon-style mustard, or a few drops of hot pepper sauce. You can also grill a tomato slice along with the mushroom, and add onions, sprouts, or field greens.

1 portobello mushroom

1/2 toasted English muffin or other bread

Pinch salt

Pinch black pepper

Desired vegetables (optional)

1. Preheat the broiler. Place the mushroom and any vegetables you wish to grill on a small baking sheet. Broil 2 inches from the heat about 3 minutes on each side or until the mushroom has shrunk slightly, exuded its juice, and begun to brown.
2. Serve on a toasted English muffin half and garnish as desired.

Preparation Time:
2 minutes

Serves 1

Exchanges

1 Starch

1 Vegetable

Calories 94

Total Fat 1 g

Saturated Fat 0 g

Calories from Fat 9

Cholesterol 0 mg

Sodium 136 mg

Carbohydrate 18 g

Dietary Fiber 2 g

Sugars 3 g

Protein 4 g

Preparation Time:
6 minutes

Serves 1

Quick Fajitas

With this quick-as-a-wink recipe, you can easily create restaurant-style fajitas at home. If you want to double or triple the recipe, use a larger skillet.

1/2 cup frozen mixed pepper and onion stir-fry
1 oz cooked diced turkey breast meat or shrimp
1 6-in low-fat flour tortilla
1–2 Tbsp mild or medium salsa

1. Coat a medium nonstick skillet with nonstick spray. Add the pepper and onion mixture and turkey or shrimp and cook over medium-high heat, stirring frequently, until the onions are softened, about 2 minutes.
2. Place the tortilla on a small plate. Spoon the pepper mixture over the tortilla. Add the salsa. Place the tortilla in the pan and reduce the heat to medium-low. Cover the skillet and cook 1 minute, until the tortilla is heated.
3. Fold the tortilla in half and serve.

Exchanges

1 Starch

1 Vegetable

1 Very Lean Meat

Calories 126

Total Fat 0 g

Saturated Fat 0 g

Calories from Fat 3

Cholesterol 23 mg

Sodium 303 mg

Carbohydrate 20 g

Dietary Fiber 2 g

Sugars 2 g

Protein 12 g

Middle Eastern Sandwich

Capture the flavors of the Middle East in this quick and tasty sandwich.

1/2 cup frozen mixed pepper and onion stir-fry

3 Tbsp chopped fresh tomato

1 Tbsp dark raisins

1 garlic clove, minced

Pinch dried thyme leaves

Pinch cinnamon

1 small whole-wheat pita bread, cut in half

1. In a medium nonstick skillet coated with nonstick spray, combine the pepper-onion mixture, tomato, raisins, garlic, thyme, and cinnamon. Stir to mix well. Cook over medium heat, stirring occasionally with a wooden spoon, until the onions are softened, about 2 to 3 minutes.
2. Divide mixture evenly in pita pockets and serve.

Preparation Time:
5 minutes

Serves 2

Serving Size:
1 pita bread half

Exchanges

1 Starch

1 Vegetable

Calories 96

Total Fat 1 g

Saturated Fat 0 g

Calories from Fat 7

Cholesterol 0 mg

Sodium 71 mg

Carbohydrate 21 g

Dietary Fiber 2 g

Sugars 6 g

Protein 3 g

Preparation Time: 20 minutes

Serves 11

Serving Size: 1 Tbsp and 1/2 oz bread

Exchanges

1 Starch

1/2 Polyunsaturated Fat

Calories 104

Total Fat 2 g

Saturated Fat 0 g

Calories from Fat 21

Cholesterol 0 mg

Sodium 118 mg

Carbohydrate 17 g

Dietary Fiber 3 g

Sugars 3 g

Protein 4 g

Falafel

Imported from the Middle East, falafel is a patty made of chickpeas and sesame butter and is traditionally deep-fried. However, I like it even better in this baked version.

1 15-oz can chickpeas (garbanzo beans), rinsed and drained

2 Tbsp tahini (sesame butter)

2 Tbsp liquid egg substitute

2 Tbsp minced green onion tops

2 garlic cloves, minced

1 tsp cumin

1/2 tsp turmeric

1/4 tsp salt, or to taste (optional)

1/8 tsp black pepper

1 small onion, chopped

1 medium tomato, chopped

1/2 cup shredded lettuce

1 small cucumber, seeded and chopped

Pita pockets, cut into halves or wedges

1. Preheat the oven to 400 degrees. In a food processor container fitted with a steel blade, process the chickpeas until ground, stopping and scraping down sides of container if necessary. (Or mash by hand.)
2. Transfer to a medium bowl, and add the tahini, egg substitute, green onion, garlic, cumin, turmeric, salt (if desired), and pepper. Stir to mix well.

3. Spray a large baking sheet with nonstick spray coating. Drop mixture by rounded tablespoonfuls onto baking sheet, flattening each portion and shaping into a patty with fingers. Bake on the center oven rack 5 minutes. Turn with a spatula. Bake an additional 4 to 5 minutes until cooked through.
4. Serve in pita pockets with onion, tomato, lettuce, and cucumber. Falafel will keep in the refrigerator 2 to 3 days and can be reheated quickly in the microwave or toaster oven on a small sheet of aluminum foil. They can also be frozen on a cookie sheet, transferred to a plastic bag, and kept in the freezer for several weeks.

Preparation Time: 15 minutes

Serves 6

Serving Size: 1 mini pita

Eggplant Mini-Pita Pocket Sandwiches

These vegetarian mini-pita sandwiches make a particularly nice warm-weather snack.

1 medium (about 1 lb) eggplant, halved lengthwise

1 medium onion, peeled, halved, and lightly rubbed with olive oil

2 medium garlic cloves, peeled and minced

1/4 cup finely minced parsley

1/4 cup plain fat-free yogurt

1/4 tsp salt, or to taste (optional)

1/4 tsp black pepper, or to taste

1 Tbsp olive oil

1–2 tsp fresh lemon juice, or to taste

6 mini onion-flavored or plain pita pockets (4-inch diameter)

1/4 cup each coarsely chopped tomato and peeled cucumber, mixed

1. Preheat the oven to 450 degrees. Line a large rimmed baking sheet with foil. Lightly spray the foil with nonstick spray coating.
2. Lay the eggplant and onion cut-side down on the foil. Roast for 20 to 25 minutes, or until the eggplant halves are just tender when pierced with a fork.
3. Let the vegetables stand until cool enough to handle. Remove the skin from the eggplant. Chop the eggplant and onion fine enough to form a rough puree.

Exchanges

1 Starch

2 Vegetable

1/2 Monounsaturated Fat

Calories 140

Total Fat 3 g

Saturated Fat 1 g

Calories from Fat 27

Cholesterol 0 mg

Sodium 173 mg

Carbohydrate 25 g

Dietary Fiber 3 g

Sugars 6 g

Protein 4 g

4. Turn out into a bowl. Stir in the garlic, parsley, yogurt, salt (if desired), pepper, oil, and lemon juice. Cover and refrigerate at least 1/2 hour and up to 3 to 4 days, if desired.
5. To serve, stuff a pocket with eggplant filling, then top with a generous tablespoon of tomato-cucumber mixture. Makes enough filling for 6 mini pita pockets. Leftover filling and tomato-cucumber mixture can be covered and refrigerated for 2 to 3 days.

Preparation Time: 5 minutes

Serves 1

Pepper and Onion Quesadilla

You'll love the crunch and taste appeal of the vegetables added to this quesadilla.

1/2 cup frozen mixed pepper and onion stir-fry
1 6-in low-fat flour tortilla
2 Tbsp grated reduced-fat Cheddar cheese
1–2 Tbsp mild or medium salsa (optional)

1. Coat a medium nonstick skillet with nonstick spray coating. Add the pepper and onion mixture and cook over medium-high heat, stirring frequently, until onions are softened, about 2 minutes.
2. Push the pepper and onion mixture to the side of the pan. Add the tortilla. Scoop up the pepper and onion mixture and arrange it evenly over the tortilla. Sprinkle with the cheese. Reduce heat to medium low. Cover skillet and cook until cheese is melted, 2 to 3 minutes.
3. If desired, spoon salsa over the melted cheese. Fold the tortilla and serve.

Exchanges

1 Starch

1 Vegetable

1/2 Saturated Fat

Calories 127

Total Fat 3 g

Saturated Fat 2 g

Calories from Fat 28

Cholesterol 10 mg

Sodium 342 mg

Carbohydrate 19 g

Dietary Fiber 2 g

Sugars 2 g

Protein 8 g

Tuna Melts

This tasty tuna melt starts with the easy tuna salad on page 12.

1 recipe tuna salad (page 12)

3 Tbsp grated sharp Cheddar cheese

3 whole-wheat or oat bran English muffin halves

1. Divide the tuna salad equally among the English muffin halves, spreading it out over the muffin surface.
2. Sprinkle the cheese on top of the tuna mixture, dividing evenly. Toast until cheese is melted.

Preparation Time:
8 minutes

Serves 3

Serving Size:
1 tuna melt

Exchanges

1 Starch

1 Lean Meat

Calories 130

Total Fat 4 g

Saturated Fat 1 g

Calories from Fat 36

Cholesterol 14 mg

Sodium 256 mg

Carbohydrate 14 g

Dietary Fiber 2 g

Sugars 2 g

Protein 10 g

Preparation Time: 10 minutes

Serves 1

Turkey and Tomato Wrap

A little turkey goes a long way in this quick wrap. And fresh basil really does make a difference in the taste. If it's unavailable, you could substitute dried basil.

1 6-in low-fat flour tortilla
2 tsp reduced-fat mayonnaise
2 slices deli-style fat-free roasted turkey breast
2 Tbsp chopped fresh tomato
1 Tbsp chopped fresh basil leaves (or 1/8 tsp dried basil)

1. Lay the tortilla flat on a small plate. Spread with the mayonnaise. Lay the turkey slices on the tortilla. Sprinkle the tortilla with the tomato and basil.
2. Roll the tortilla and turkey around the tomato-basil filling. Eat like a rolled sandwich.

Exchanges

1 Starch

1 Lean Meat

Calories 147
Total Fat 3 g
Saturated Fat 1 g
Calories from Fat 30
Cholesterol 27 mg
Sodium 297 mg
Carbohydrate 19 g
Dietary Fiber 1 g
Sugars 1 g
Protein 12 g

Vegetable Wrap

Preparation Time: 5 minutes

Serves 2

Serving Size: 1 wrap

You can make the vegetable mixture, serve half of it in a tortilla, and save the rest in the refrigerator for the next day. If you like, substitute large lettuce or romaine leaves for the tortillas.

1/2 cup peeled, chopped cucumber

1/4 cup chopped sweet red or green pepper

2 large pitted black olives, chopped

1 large plum tomato, chopped

2 Tbsp thinly sliced green onion tops

1/4 cup reduced-fat sour cream

1/2 tsp Italian seasoning

2 small low-fat flour tortillas

1. In a small bowl, combine the cucumber, pepper, olives, tomato, and green onion. Stir to mix. Stir in the sour cream and the Italian seasoning.
2. Divide the filling evenly between the two flour tortillas, laying the mixture in a line down the center of each. Roll each tortilla around the filling. Serve immediately.

Exchanges

1 Starch

1 Vegetable

1 Fat

Calories 161

Total Fat 5 g

Saturated Fat 1 g

Calories from Fat 48

Cholesterol 10 mg

Sodium 211 mg

Carbohydrate 24 g

Dietary Fiber 3 g

Sugars 5 g

Protein 4 g

Preparation Time: 8 minutes

Serves 2

Serving Size: 1 wrap

Exchanges

1 Starch

1 Vegetable

1 Monounsaturated Fat

Calories 170

Total Fat 7 g

Saturated Fat 1 g

Calories from Fat 64

Cholesterol 0 mg

Sodium 169 mg

Carbohydrate 23 g

Dietary Fiber 3 g

Sugars 4 g

Protein 5 g

Pan-Grilled Vegetable Wrap

I've used a little olive oil in this recipe because it helps cook the vegetables and improves their texture. If you'd like, you can substitute nonstick spray coating. However, the vegetables will take longer to cook.

2 tsp olive oil

1 cup frozen mixed pepper and onion stir-fry

3/4 cup chopped broccoli or cauliflower florets

1/2 cup chopped zucchini

1 garlic clove, minced

Generous 1/2 tsp Italian seasoning

1/8 tsp salt (optional)

Pinch black pepper

2 small low-fat flour tortillas

1. Place the olive oil in a medium nonstick skillet. Add the onion and pepper mixture, broccoli, zucchini, garlic, Italian seasoning, salt (if desired), and pepper. Cook over medium-high heat, stirring frequently, until the vegetables are tender-crisp and begin to brown slightly, about 4 to 5 minutes.
2. To warm the tortillas, transfer the vegetables to a small plate. Lower the heat and place each tortilla, one at a time, in the skillet for 30 to 40 seconds.
3. Divide the vegetables between the tortillas, wrapping the tortilla around the filling. Serve immediately.

South of the Border Pizza

Preparation Time:
3 minutes

Serves 2

Serving Size:
1 muffin half

Say olé to this easy pizza variation made with salsa and Cheddar cheese and served on an English muffin half.

1/3 cup frozen mixed pepper and onion stir-fry

Scant 1/4 cup mild or medium salsa

1/4 cup shredded reduced-fat Cheddar cheese

1 whole-wheat English muffin

1. In a medium nonstick skillet coated with nonstick spray coating, cook the onion and pepper mixture over medium heat, stirring frequently, until the onion is tender, about 4 to 6 minutes.
2. Meanwhile, divide the salsa evenly between the English muffin halves, and spread it evenly over each half. Sprinkle the cheese evenly over the two halves. Toast the muffin halves in a toaster oven until the cheese melts.
3. When the onion and pepper mixture is done, top the pizza halves with the pepper mixture, dividing it evenly.

Exchanges

1 Starch

1 Medium Fat Meat

Calories 165

Total Fat 7 g

Saturated Fat 4 g

Calories from Fat 61

Cholesterol 20 mg

Sodium 426 mg

Carbohydrate 15 g

Dietary Fiber 2 g

Sugars 4 g

Protein 12 g

Egg Salad Sandwich

Preparation Time: 6 minutes

Serves 2

Serving Size: 1/3 cup egg salad with 1 bread slice

If you love egg salad but have cut it from your meal plan because of the cholesterol, try this zippy recipe, which discards half of the egg yolks. With all of the taste of traditional egg salad and far less fat, it's one of my favorite sandwiches.

2 hard-cooked large eggs, cooled under running water

1 Tbsp fat-free sour cream

2 tsp sweet pickle relish

2 tsp reduced-fat mayonnaise

1/4 tsp Dijon-style mustard

Pinch salt (optional)

1/4 cup finely chopped celery

2 slices reduced-fat whole-wheat bread

Paprika for garnish (optional)

1. Cut each egg in half. Carefully remove the yolks. Discard one yolk.
2. In a small bowl, mash the remaining egg yolk. Add the sour cream, pickle relish, mayonnaise, mustard, and salt (if desired). Stir to mix well. Stir in the celery. Chop the egg whites and stir them into the yolk mixture.
3. Spread the mixture on each slice of bread. Serve as open-faced sandwiches. If desired, garnish with a light sprinkling of paprika.

Exchanges

1 Starch

1 Medium Fat Meat

Calories 148

Total Fat 7 g

Saturated Fat 2 g

Calories from Fat 62

Cholesterol 215 mg

Sodium 296 mg

Carbohydrate 14 g

Dietary Fiber 3 g

Sugars 4 g

Protein 9 g

Quick Turkey Salad Sandwich

Roasted turkey breast is wonderfully low in fat but high in flavor. Here it's spiced up with red onion and balsamic vinegar. Instead of serving the turkey salad on an English muffin half, you could roll it in a flour tortilla.

3/4 oz roasted turkey breast

1 Tbsp fat-free sour cream

1 tsp reduced-fat mayonnaise

1/2 Tbsp chopped red onion

1/4 tsp balsamic vinegar

Pinch of salt and pepper

Pinch of dried rosemary leaves, or 1/4 tsp fresh rosemary

1/2 oat bran English muffin, toasted

1. Cut the turkey into very small bite-sized pieces. Set aside.
2. In a small bowl, stir together the sour cream, mayonnaise, onion, vinegar, salt, pepper, and rosemary. Stir in the turkey.
3. Mound the mixture on an English muffin half.

Preparation Time: 5 minutes

Serves 1

Exchanges

1 Starch

1 Very Lean Meat

Calories 123

Total Fat 2 g

Saturated Fat 0 g

Calories from Fat 21

Cholesterol 19 mg

Sodium 181 mg

Carbohydrate 16 g

Dietary Fiber 2 g

Sugars 4 g

Protein 10 g

Just For Fun

Here are some recipes I wanted to include in *The Diabetes Snack Munch Nibble Nosh Book* but simply couldn't classify under any other heading. Included are a number of real treats, such as Better Deviled Eggs, that go a long way toward reducing the fat and cholesterol in traditional snack and picnic favorites.

Two recipes, Parmesan Triangles and Asian Triangles, are made with wonton wrappers, which are sold in the produce department of most large supermarkets. They're fat free and crisp up nicely when garnished and baked in the oven.

Pico de Gallo

Preparation Time:
20 minutes

Serves 20

Serving Size:
2 Tbsp

Pico de gallo is simply the Spanish name for fresh salsa. The name means "rooster's beak" because salsa can have quite a bite, depending on the chilis used. In summer, I make this dip with ripe tomatoes. In winter, I use plum tomatoes. If you dislike the distinctive taste of cilantro, you can leave it out. Be sure to wash your hands thoroughly after handling hot chili peppers, as they can leave an oily residue on your skin that can irritate your eyes.

2 fresh, mild jalapeño chili peppers, seeds and membranes removed, finely chopped

2 cups diced fresh tomatoes

1/2 cup thinly sliced green onions, white and green parts

2 Tbsp chopped cilantro

Grated zest of 1 lime

1–2 Tbsp fresh lime juice, or to taste

1/4 tsp salt, or to taste (optional)

1. In a medium bowl, combine the chilis, tomatoes, onions, cilantro, lime zest, lime juice, and salt (if desired). Stir to mix well.
2. Serve immediately with fat-free tortilla chips, or cover and refrigerate 3 to 4 hours before serving. Pico de gallo will keep in the refrigerator 3 to 4 days.

Exchange

Free

Calories 7

Total Fat 0 g

Saturated Fat 0 g

Calories from Fat 1

Cholesterol 0 mg

Sodium 2 mg

Carbohydrate 2 g

Dietary Fiber 0 g

Sugars 1 g

Protein 0 g

Preparation Time: 15 minutes

Serves 28

Serving Size: 2 Tbsp

Black Bean Salsa

Serve this fresh and spicy salsa with fat-free tortilla chips. Be sure to wash your hands well after handling hot chili peppers, since the oily residue left on your skin can cause eye irritation.

- 1 large tomato, chopped
- 1/4 cup thinly sliced green onion tops
- 1/2 sweet red or green pepper, seeded and chopped
- 1 medium jalapeño chili pepper, seeds and membrane removed, chopped
- 2 tsp olive oil
- 2 tsp lemon juice
- 1/4 tsp dried oregano leaves
- 1 large garlic clove, minced
- 1/4 tsp salt, or to taste (optional)
- 1 3/4 cups cooked black beans, or 1 15-oz can black beans, rinsed and well drained

1. In a medium bowl, combine the tomato, green onions, sweet pepper, hot pepper, olive oil, lemon juice, oregano, garlic, and salt (if desired). Stir to mix well.
2. Carefully stir in the black beans. Serve at once, or cover and refrigerate 1 hour or up to 24 hours before serving.
3. The salsa will keep for 4 to 5 days in the refrigerator. Serve with fat-free tortilla chips.

Exchange

Free

Calories 20

Total Fat 0 g

Saturated Fat 0 g

Calories from Fat 4

Cholesterol 0 mg

Sodium 1 mg

Carbohydrate 3 g

Dietary Fiber 1 g

Sugars 1 g

Protein 1 g

Better Deviled Eggs

This is a healthier version of a traditional favorite.

2 hard-cooked large eggs, cooled under running water

2 tsp fat-free sour cream

1 tsp sweet pickle relish

1 tsp reduced-fat mayonnaise

1/8–1/4 tsp Dijon-style mustard

Pinch salt (optional)

2 Tbsp finely chopped celery

1. Cut each egg in half. Carefully remove the yolks. Discard one yolk.
2. In a custard cup, mash the remaining egg yolk. Add the sour cream, pickle relish, mayonnaise, mustard, and salt (if desired). Stir to mix well. Stir in the celery.
3. Serve at once, or cover and refrigerate. Deviled eggs will keep in the refrigerator 1 to 2 days.

Preparation Time: 3 minutes

Serves 2

Serving Size: 1 egg

Exchanges

1 Lean Meat

Calories 64

Total Fat 3 g

Saturated Fat 1 g

Calories from Fat 30

Cholesterol 107 mg

Sodium 121 mg

Carbohydrate 3 g

Dietary Fiber 0 g

Sugars 2 g

Protein 5 g

Preparation Time: 15 minutes

Serves 16

Serving Size: 2 Tbsp

Easy Corn Relish

Serve this corn relish on fat-free crackers or on a whole-wheat or oat bran English muffin half.

2 cups frozen corn kernels, cooked according to package directions

2/3 cup chili sauce

1 celery stalk, chopped

1/2 red bell pepper, seeded and chopped

2 Tbsp chopped chives or thinly sliced green onion tops

1 tsp olive oil

1/4 tsp dried thyme leaves

1 garlic clove, minced

1. Cool the cooked corn in a colander under cold running water. Drain.
2. In a medium bowl, combine the chili sauce, celery, red pepper, chives, oil, thyme, and garlic. Stir to mix well. Stir in the corn.
3. Serve at room temperature, or cover and refrigerate. Relish will keep in the refrigerator for 3 to 4 days.

Exchanges

1/2 Starch

Calories 32

Total Fat 0 g

Saturated Fat 0 g

Calories from Fat 4

Cholesterol 0 mg

Sodium 138 mg

Carbohydrate 7 g

Dietary Fiber 1 g

Sugars 2 g

Protein 1 g

Strawberry-Peach Cooler

This easy, refreshing fruit shake has become one of my summer favorites. I love the natural tartness of the fruit combination, but if you'd prefer a sweeter drink, add a small amount of artificial sweetener to taste. The partially frozen fruit gives the shake its icy texture.

1 cup dry-pack unsweetened frozen strawberries

2/3 cup dry-pack unsweetened frozen peaches

3/4 cup orange juice

1. In a 2-cup measure or similar microwave-safe bowl, combine the strawberries and peaches. Cover with wax paper, and microwave on high power 45 seconds to 1 minute to thaw the fruit slightly. The fruit should be icy but not hard. Working with a small knife in the measuring cup, cut each peach slice in half.
2. Transfer the peaches and strawberries to a blender container. Add the orange juice. Blend on low power to combine. Then increase power to high and continue to blend until the peaches are completely pureed, at least 1 1/2 minutes.

Preparation Time: 6 minutes

Serves 2

Serving Size: 1 cup

Exchanges

2 Fruit

Calories 105

Total Fat 0 g

Saturated Fat 0 g

Calories from Fat 2

Cholesterol 0 mg

Sodium 2 mg

Carbohydrate 26 g

Dietary Fiber 3 g

Sugars 23 g

Protein 2 g

Preparation Time: 6 minutes

Serves 2

Serving Size: 1 generous cup

Mango Lassi

Lassi, a tart, cooling yogurt drink, is a treat I've learned to enjoy in Indian restaurants. Happily, it's easy to make at home. Mango is one of the traditional fruit flavors used.

1 ripe mango

1 8-oz carton reduced-fat yogurt

1/2 cup very cold water

1. Remove the flesh from the mango, discarding the skin and seed. You should have about 1 cup of mango.
2. Combine the mango, yogurt, and water in a blender container. Blend on medium speed until well combined and smooth. Serve at once.
3. Leftover lassi can be tightly covered and kept in the refrigerator for 24 hours. Stir before serving.

Exchanges

1 Fruit

1/2 Reduced Fat Milk

Calories 128

Total Fat 2 g

Saturated Fat 1 g

Calories from Fat 20

Cholesterol 10 mg

Sodium 88 mg

Carbohydrate 23 g

Dietary Fiber 2 g

Sugars 21 g

Protein 7 g

Banana-Strawberry Shake

Be sure to use a very ripe banana in this tart and refreshing fruit shake.

1 very ripe banana, cut into large chunks

1 cup dry-pack unsweetened frozen strawberries

1 cup low-fat (1%) milk

In a blender container, combine the banana, strawberries, and milk. Blend on medium speed until the strawberries are completely pureed and the shake is smooth. Serve at once.

Preparation Time:
4 minutes

Serves 2

Serving Size:
1 1/4 cups

Exchanges

1 Fruit

1/2 Reduced Fat Milk

Calories 117

Total Fat 2 g

Saturated Fat 1 g

Calories from Fat 14

Cholesterol 5 mg

Sodium 64 mg

Carbohydrate 23 g

Dietary Fiber 3 g

Sugars 17 g

Protein 5 g

Preparation Time: 13 minutes

Serves 14

Serving Size: 1/2 cup

Exchanges

1 Starch

1/2 Fruit

1/2 Polyunsaturated Fat

Calories 123

Total Fat 2 g

Saturated Fat 0 g

Calories from Fat 19

Cholesterol 0 mg

Sodium 172 mg

Carbohydrate 26 g

Dietary Fiber 3 g

Sugars 8 g

Protein 2 g

Screws and Bolts

I fell in love with this homemade snack mix the first time I tasted it at a friend's house after school. For me, it was an exotic treat, since my mother bought all of her crunchy snacks from the grocery store. This version retains the intense flavor of the original.

1/4 cup reduced-fat tubstyle margarine (4.5 g fat/T)

2 Tbsp Worcestershire sauce

1 tsp chili powder

1 tsp paprika

Pinch garlic powder

1/2 tsp salt, or to taste (optional)

3–4 drops hot pepper sauce

3 cups unsalted thin pretzels (large pieces broken up before measuring)

2 cups wheat squares cereal

2 cups bran squares cereal

1 cup toasted oat O's cereal

1/2 cup raisins

1/2 cup chopped dried apricots

1. Preheat the oven to 300 degrees. Coat a large, shallow baking pan with nonstick cooking spray and set aside.
2. In a 1-cup measure or similar small microwave-safe bowl, mix together the margarine, Worcestershire sauce, chili powder, paprika, garlic powder, salt (if desired), and hot pepper sauce. Cover with wax paper, and microwave on

high power about 1 minute or until margarine is almost melted. Stir to combine ingredients. Set aside.

3. In the baking pan, combine the pretzels, wheat squares, bran squares, and toasted oat O's. Slowly drizzle the margarine mixture over the cereal mixture, lifting and stirring very well to coat the cereal and pretzels as evenly as possible.
4. Bake for 25 minutes, stirring twice to prevent mixture on the bottom from burning, or until mixture is crisp. Cool the pan on a wire rack. Stir in the raisins and apricots while the mixture is still warm.
5. Cool before serving. Store in an air-tight container. The mixture will keep for up to a week at room temperature.

Easy Cheese Popcorn

Preparation Time: 6 minutes

Serves 10

Serving Size: 1 cup

Popcorn makes a great snack. Here's a cheese popcorn that won't bust your fat budget.

10 cups air-popped or low-fat microwave popcorn

3 oz (about 3/4 cup) shredded reduced-fat Cheddar cheese

1. Preheat the oven to 375 degrees. Remove any unpopped kernels from the popcorn, and spread the popcorn on a large cookie sheet with sides. Popcorn should cover the pan bottom in a single layer, with as few as possible spaces in between kernels.
2. Slowly, sprinkle the cheese over the popcorn, being careful that the cheese remains on the kernels. Bake for 3 to 4 minutes or until the cheese has melted onto the popcorn. Loosen any stuck cheese from the bottom of the pan with a broad spatula. Cool the popcorn in the pan on a wire rack. Serve immediately. Popcorn will keep for 2 to 3 days in an airtight container.

Exchanges

1/2 Starch

1/2 Saturated Fat

Calories 58

Total Fat 2 g

Saturated Fat 1 g

Calories from Fat 19

Cholesterol 6 mg

Sodium 69 mg

Carbohydrate 6 g

Dietary Fiber 1 g

Sugars 0 g

Protein 4 g

Mustard Pretzels

These tangy pretzels make a great snack. If you like a spicier pretzel, add a bit more mustard.

6 cups small pretzels (about 3/16 inch in diameter)

3 Tbsp prepared mustard

1 Tbsp mild or strong honey

1/2 Tbsp cider vinegar

1/4 tsp dry mustard

1. Preheat the oven to 400 degrees. Spray a large baking pan with nonstick spray coating. Arrange the pretzels in the pan.
2. In a small bowl, stir together the prepared mustard, honey, vinegar, and dry mustard. Slowly pour the mixture over the pretzels, stirring to coat.
3. Spread out the pretzels so that they are in 1 or 2 layers. Bake for 8 to 10 minutes, stirring once, or until the pretzels begin to brown. Cool in the pan on a wire rack until they begin to crisp. The pretzels will keep at room temperature for 1 to 2 weeks.

Preparation Time:
8 minutes

Serves 6

Serving Size:
1 cup

Exchanges

1 1/2 Starch

Calories 124

Total Fat 1 g

Saturated Fat 0 g

Calories from Fat 11

Cholesterol 0 mg

Sodium 575 mg

Carbohydrate 26 g

Dietary Fiber 1 g

Sugars 4 g

Protein 3 g

Garlic-Parmesan Rolls

Preparation Time: 3 minutes

Serves 2

Serving Size: 1/2 roll

If you like garlic bread, try these crispy rolls. It's most convenient to make them in the toaster oven, but you can also use the conventional oven. To speed the preparation of this recipe, I use prechopped garlic, available in the produce section of the supermarket.

1 whole-wheat or mixed-grain dinner roll (about 1 3/4 oz)

2 tsp reduced-fat tubstyle margarine (4.5 g fat/T)

1/4–1/2 tsp chopped garlic, or to taste

Pinch basil

2 tsp grated Parmesan cheese

1. If using the conventional oven, preheat to 425 degrees.
2. Cut the roll in half. Spread each half with half the margarine and half the garlic. Sprinkle on the Parmesan cheese, and press it into place with the back of a spoon.
3. If using the toaster oven, place the roll halves on the rack, and crisp until browned. Serve immediately.
4. If using the conventional oven, lay the rolls on a baking sheet and bake for about 5 minutes or until browned. Serve warm.

Exchanges

1 Starch

1/2 Fat

Calories 86

Total Fat 3 g

Saturated Fat 1 g

Calories from Fat 30

Cholesterol 3 mg

Sodium 203 mg

Carbohydrate 12 g

Dietary Fiber 2 g

Sugars 2 g

Protein 4 g

Tortilla Pinwheels

Before making these easy pinwheels, check the tortilla nutrition labels. While some tortillas are quite high in fat, others have almost none.

1 Tbsp fat-free cream cheese

2 Tbsp shredded reduced-fat Cheddar cheese

2 Tbsp mild salsa

1 Tbsp chopped green onion tops

1/8 tsp chili powder

1 6-in low-fat flour tortilla

1. In a small bowl, stir together the cream cheese and Cheddar cheese with a fork until the Cheddar is incorporated. Stir in the salsa, green onion, and chili powder.
2. Spread the mixture evenly on the tortilla. Roll up and cut off the two ends. Cut tortilla into 4 pieces and serve.

Preparation Time: 10 minutes

Serves 2

Serving Size: 2 pieces

Exchanges

1/2 Starch

1 Very Lean Meat

Calories 70

Total Fat 2 g

Saturated Fat 1 g

Calories from Fat 14

Cholesterol 6 mg

Sodium 258 mg

Carbohydrate 10 g

Dietary Fiber 1 g

Sugars 1 g

Protein 5 g

Preparation Time:
5 minutes

Serves 1

Nachos

Here's a quick recipe to use when you get a hankering for nachos. They take no time at all in the conventional oven or the toaster oven.

4 large fat-free tortilla chips

2 Tbsp reduced-fat Cheddar cheese

3 Tbsp mild or medium low-sodium or regular salsa

1 1/2 Tbsp fat-free sour cream

1. If using the conventional oven, preheat to 400 degrees. Arrange tortilla chips (concave side up) on a medium baking sheet. Sprinkle evenly with the cheese. Divide the salsa among the chips. Bake just until cheese melts, about 2 to 3 minutes.
2. If using the toaster oven, arrange chips on a sheet of aluminum foil. Toast until cheese just melts.
3. Remove from the oven and add a dollop of sour cream to each chip.

Exchanges

1 Starch

1 Very Lean Meat

Calories 109

Total Fat 3 g

Saturated Fat 2 g

Calories from Fat 30

Cholesterol 10 mg

Sodium 295 mg

Carbohydrate 13 g

Dietary Fiber 2 g

Sugars 6 g

Protein 8 g

Asian Triangles

Preparation Time: 8 minutes

Serves 6

Serving Size: 4 pieces

These tangy triangles are fun to make and fun to eat.

1 Tbsp smooth peanut butter

1/2 Tbsp lite soy sauce

1 tsp water

1/2 tsp Asian sesame oil

4 tsp rice or white vinegar

1/4 tsp ginger

2–3 drops hot pepper sauce

12 wonton wrappers, cut in half to form triangles

1. Preheat the oven to 400 degrees. Spray a large baking sheet with nonstick spray coating. Set aside.
2. In a small microwave-safe bowl, combine the peanut butter, soy sauce, water, oil, vinegar, ginger, and hot pepper sauce. Microwave 20 to 30 seconds to warm the mixture so that peanut butter will easily combine with the other ingredients. With a small wire whisk, whisk until well combined.
3. Arrange the wonton wrappers on the baking sheet in a single layer. With your finger, brush the mixture over the top of the wonton triangles.
4. Bake for 3 to 5 minutes, or until the triangles have crisped. Cool in the pan on a wire rack, or serve warm. Triangles will keep for up to a week in an airtight container.

Exchanges

1/2 Starch

1/2 Fat

Calories 54

Total Fat 2 g

Saturated Fat 0 g

Calories from Fat 17

Cholesterol 2 mg

Sodium 131 mg

Carbohydrate 8 g

Dietary Fiber 1 g

Sugars 1 g

Protein 2 g

Preparation Time:
8 minutes

Serves 10

Serving Size:
5 pieces

Parmesan Triangles

Try these crispy Parmesan snacks the next time your friends drop in.

1 Tbsp olive oil

1 Tbsp water

1 garlic clove, minced

1 tsp Italian seasoning

25 wonton wrappers, cut in half to form triangles

2 Tbsp grated Parmesan cheese

1. Preheat the oven to 400 degrees. Spray a large baking sheet with nonstick spray coating. Set aside.
2. In a small bowl, stir together the oil, water, garlic, and Italian seasoning.
3. Set the wonton wrappers on the baking sheet in a single layer.
4. With your finger, spread the oil mixture over the wonton triangles. (If the mixture begins to separate, stir again.) Sprinkle with the cheese.
5. Bake for 3 to 4 minutes until the triangles have crisped. Cool in pan on a wire rack, or serve warm. Triangles will keep for up to a week in an airtight container.

Exchanges

1/2 Starch

1/2 Monounsaturated Fat

Calories 61

Total Fat 2 g

Saturated Fat 1 g

Calories from Fat 18

Cholesterol 4 mg

Sodium 111 mg

Carbohydrate 9 g

Dietary Fiber 1 g

Sugars 0 g

Protein 2 g

The Bake Shop

The savory dishes in this chapter are served hot from the oven. Included is a corn bread that can be served as a snack any time or even for breakfast. I've also developed an easy dough you can use for homemade pizza or calzone, which are Italian baked turnovers. It's fun to make your own dough, but if you like, you can save time by purchasing an unbaked pizza crust.

Preparation Time: 25 minutes (crust only)

Serves 9

Serving Size: 1 oz

Exchanges

1 Starch

1/2 Monounsaturated Fat

Calories 94

Total Fat 2 g

Saturated Fat 0 g

Calories from Fat 15

Cholesterol 0 mg

Sodium 195 mg

Carbohydrate 17 g

Dietary Fiber 1 g

Sugars 1 g

Protein 3 g

Pizza or Calzone Crust

Here's an easy dough that can be used for either pizza or calzone. You can make it in a food processor or knead it by hand. Water temperature is important for good results. If the water is too hot, it will kill the yeast. If it's too cold, the yeast won't make the dough rise. Test the water-oil mixture with a candy thermometer before adding it to the flour-yeast mixture.

1 3/4 cups all-purpose white flour

1 package quick-rising yeast

3/4 tsp salt

1/2 tsp sugar

2/3 cup water (125–130 degrees F)

1 Tbsp olive oil

1. In a food processor container fitted with a steel blade, combine the flour, yeast, salt, and sugar. Pulse to mix. Combine hot water and olive oil and test temperature. With food processor on, gradually add the water-oil mixture through the feed tube. Process until the dough forms a ball, 5 to 10 seconds. Then process for 1 minute longer to knead. Remove the dough from processor. If it seems sticky, work in 2 or 3 tsp of flour.
2. To mix by hand, combine the flour, yeast, salt, and sugar in a medium bowl. Combine the hot water and the oil and test temperature. With a large spoon, stir in the water-oil mixture and mix in. Knead by hand until a smooth dough is formed, about 3 to 5 minutes. If the dough seems sticky, work in 2 or 3 additional tsp of flour.

3. Turn dough out onto a lightly floured board. Spray plastic wrap with nonstick spray, cover dough, and let rise 15 minutes.
4. Preheat the oven to 425 degrees. Spray a large baking sheet or pizza pan with nonstick spray. Lightly sprinkle with cornmeal, if desired. Transfer the dough to the pan. Stretch and shape the dough by hand and/or with a rolling pin into a 12- or 13-inch circle or an 11- by 14-inch rectangle. Add additional ingredients for pizza or calzone from recipes on pages 60, 62, 64, and 66. Bake for 15 to 17 minutes on center oven rack or until crust is lightly browned.

Preparation Time: 20 minutes

Serves 9

Serving Size: 1 piece

Spinach, Red Onion, and Cheese Pizza

If you like white pizza (with no tomato sauce), try this cheese and spinach version. It can be made with the dough on page 58 or on a store-bought pizza crust.

1 homemade or store-bought pizza crust (see recipe, p. 58)

1 1/2 cups loose-leaf, dry-pack frozen spinach

1/4 cup chopped red onion

1/2 cup fat-free ricotta cheese

1 1/4 tsp Italian seasoning

1 garlic clove, minced

2–3 drops hot pepper sauce

1/3 cup crumbled feta cheese

2 Tbsp grated Parmesan cheese

1. Preheat the oven to 425 degrees. Spray a large baking sheet or pizza pan with nonstick spray. Lightly sprinkle with cornmeal, if desired. Set aside.
2. If making the crust, transfer the dough to the pan. Stretch and shape the dough by hand and/or with rolling pin into a 12- or 13-inch circle or 11- by 14-inch rectangle. If using store-bought crust, place it on the pan.
3. Place the spinach and red onion in a small microwave-safe bowl, cover with wax paper, and microwave on defrost power for 2 to 3 minutes, or until the spinach is thawed and the onion is softened.

Exchanges

1 Starch

1 Vegetable

1/2 Fat

Calories 133

Total Fat 3 g

Saturated Fat 1 g

Calories from Fat 29

Cholesterol 10 mg

Sodium 308 mg

Carbohydrate 20 g

Dietary Fiber 2 g

Sugars 2 g

Protein 7 g

4. Place the ricotta in a small bowl and stir in the spinach mixture, Italian seasoning, garlic, and hot pepper sauce. Spread the ricotta mixture onto the pizza dough. Sprinkle with the feta and Parmesan cheeses.
5. For homemade crust, bake for 15 to 17 minutes on center oven rack or until crust is lightly browned. For store-bought crust, bake according to package directions. Cut into 9 rectangles or wedges and serve.

Preparation Time:
20 minutes

Serves 8

Serving Size:
1 piece

Artichoke, Shrimp, and Roasted Red Pepper Pizza

Make this tasty pizza with the homemade crust on page 58, or use a store-bought pizza crust.

1 homemade or store-bought pizza crust (see recipe, p. 58)

1 cup water-packed artichoke heart quarters, well drained

1 cup pizza sauce

1 1/2 cups cooked shrimp

1/4 cup roasted red pepper, chopped

2 Tbsp grated Parmesan cheese

1. Preheat the oven to 425 degrees. Spray a large baking sheet or pizza pan with nonstick spray. Lightly sprinkle with cornmeal, if desired.
2. If making the crust, transfer the dough to the pan. Stretch and shape the dough by hand and/or with rolling pin into a 12- or 13-inch circle or 11- by 14-inch rectangle. If using store-bought crust, place it on the pan.
3. Remove and discard any coarse outer leaves from the artichoke hearts. Coarsely chop the hearts.
4. Spread the pizza sauce over the crust. Sprinkle the artichoke hearts evenly over the crust. Sprinkle on the shrimp, then the chopped pepper. Top with cheese.
5. If using homemade crust, bake for 12 to 15 minutes. If using purchased crust, bake according to package directions, or until the pizza begins to brown at edges. Cut into 9 rectangles or wedges and serve.

Exchanges

1 Starch

1 Vegetable

1 Lean Meat

Calories 164

Total Fat 3 g

Saturated Fat 1 g

Calories from Fat 29

Cholesterol 49 mg

Sodium 559 mg

Carbohydrate 24 g

Dietary Fiber 2 g

Sugars 3 g

Protein 10 g

Pizza Puffs

Here are puffy individual pizza snacks in minutes!

1 4 1/2-oz package reduced-fat refrigerator buttermilk biscuits

1 1/2 Tbsp low-sodium or regular tomato sauce

Scant 1/2 tsp Italian seasoning

1/2 Tbsp grated Parmesan cheese

1. Preheat the oven to 450 degrees. Spray a small baking sheet with nonstick spray coating. Set aside.
2. In a custard cup, mix together the tomato sauce and Italian seasoning. Set aside.
3. Open the biscuit carton and separate the biscuits. Place them on the baking sheet.
4. With a small spoon, spread the tomato sauce and seasoning mixture on the biscuits, dividing the mixture evenly. Bake in the center of the oven for 8 to 10 minutes or until golden. Serve hot.
5. Leftovers will keep 1 to 2 days in the refrigerator, tightly wrapped.

Preparation Time: 6 minutes

Serves 6

Serving Size: 1 piece

Exchanges

1/2 Starch

Calories 54

Total Fat 1 g

Saturated Fat 0 g

Calories from Fat 8

Cholesterol 1 mg

Sodium 191 mg

Carbohydrate 10 g

Dietary Fiber 0 g

Sugars 1 g

Protein 2 g

Preparation Time: 20 minutes

Serves 8

Serving Size: 1 piece

Barbecued Chicken Pizza

Barbecued chicken makes a differently delicious pizza topping. Use the homemade crust on page 58 or a store-bought crust. For the chicken, you can use leftover roast chicken or quickly cook a chicken breast in the microwave.

1 homemade or store-bought pizza crust (see recipe, p. 58)

1 8-oz can low-sodium or regular tomato sauce

1 small onion, finely chopped

1 Tbsp packed light brown sugar

1/2 tsp cider vinegar

1/2 tsp dry mustard

1/4 tsp dried thyme leaves

Pinch of cloves

1/8 tsp black pepper

2–3 drops hot pepper sauce (optional)

1/2 cup cooked chicken breast meat, cut into very small pieces

3/4 cup shredded reduced-fat Cheddar cheese

1. Preheat the oven to 400 degrees. Spray a large baking sheet or pizza pan with nonstick spray. Lightly sprinkle with cornmeal, if desired.
2. If making the crust, transfer the dough to the pan. Stretch and shape the dough by hand and/or with rolling pin into a 12- or 13-inch circle or 11- by 14-inch rectangle. If using store-bought crust, place it on the pan.

Exchanges

1 1/2 Starch

1 Meat

Calories 172

Total Fat 5 g

Saturated Fat 2 g

Calories from Fat 41

Cholesterol 15 mg

Sodium 318 mg

Carbohydrate 24 g

Dietary Fiber 1 g

Sugars 4 g

Protein 9 g

3. In a 2-cup measure or similar microwave-safe container, combine the tomato sauce, onion, brown sugar, vinegar, mustard, thyme, cloves, pepper, and hot pepper sauce (if desired). Cover with wax paper, and microwave on high power 1 1/2 to 2 minutes, until the sauce is bubbly. Stir in the chicken.
4. Spread the mixture on the pizza crust. Sprinkle with cheese. If using homemade crust, bake for 8 to 10 minutes. If using purchased crust, bake according to package directions, or until the pizza begins to brown at edges. Cut into 8 rectangles or wedges and serve.

Preparation Time: 45 minutes

Serves 9

Serving Size: 1 piece

Mini Spinach and Cheese Calzone

Calzone are Italian baked turnovers. I've used an easy dough (see recipe, page 58) and a creamy spinach and cheese filling in these.

1 homemade or store-bought pizza crust (see recipe, p. 58)

1 3/4 cups loose-leaf, dry-pack frozen spinach

3/4 cup fat-free ricotta cheese

1 1/4 cups shredded reduced-fat mozzarella cheese

3 Tbsp grated Parmesan cheese

1 1/2 tsp olive oil

1 1/4 tsp Italian seasoning

1 garlic clove, minced

Pinch nutmeg

1/8 tsp salt (optional)

2–3 drops hot pepper sauce

1 Tbsp low-fat (1%) milk (optional)

1. Preheat the oven to 375 degrees. Spray a large baking sheet or pizza pan with nonstick spray. Lightly sprinkle with cornmeal, if desired. In a large bowl, combine all remaining ingredients except the milk.
2. Divide the dough into 9 equal portions. On a lightly floured board, roll each portion of the dough into a 5-inch circle, adding additional flour to board if needed. (Hint: if the dough is difficult to roll to this diameter, roll each circle to 4 inches. Allow to rest before rolling out to full 5 inches.) While working, stack circles on a plate, covering with plastic wrap.

Exchanges

1 Starch

1 Vegetable

1 Lean Meat

Calories 170

Total Fat 5 g

Saturated Fat 2 g

Calories from Fat 42

Cholesterol 16 mg

Sodium 374 mg

Carbohydrate 20 g

Dietary Fiber 2 g

Sugars 1 g

Protein 12 g

3. For each calzone, spoon about 2 generous tablespoons of the filling mixture onto half of one dough circle, leaving 1/2 inch at the edge. Moisten the edges of the dough with water. Fold the dough in half over the filling. Seal by pressing with fork tines.
4. Transfer the calzone to the prepared baking sheet. Prick the top to allow steam to escape. For a richer appearance, brush tops of the calzone lightly with milk before baking. Bake on the center oven rack for 20 to 22 minutes or until crust is lightly browned. Let cool 3 to 4 minutes before serving.

Preparation Time: 8 minutes

Serves 10

Serving Size: 1 piece

Ham and Cheese Puffs

These puffy little ham and cheese biscuits make a great snack or appetizer.

1 7 1/2-oz package reduced-fat refrigerator buttermilk biscuits or rolls

3 Tbsp seasoned tomato sauce

2 Tbsp chopped reduced-fat ham or Canadian bacon

2 Tbsp reduced-fat shredded Cheddar cheese

1. Preheat the oven to 450 degrees. Spray a small baking sheet with nonstick spray coating. Set aside.
2. Open the biscuit carton, and separate the biscuits. Place them on the baking sheet.
3. With a small spoon, spread the tomato sauce on the biscuits, dividing the mixture evenly. Top with the ham and cheese, dividing evenly.
4. Bake in the center of the oven for 8 to 10 minutes or until golden. Serve hot. Leftovers will keep 1 to 2 days in the refrigerator, tightly wrapped.

Exchanges

1/2 Starch

Calories 59

Total Fat 1 g

Saturated Fat 0 g

Calories from Fat 10

Cholesterol 2 mg

Sodium 231 mg

Carbohydrate 10 g

Dietary Fiber 0 g

Sugars 1 g

Protein 2 g

Tex-Mex Cornbread

Preparation Time:
18 minutes

Serves 9

Serving Size:
1 square

This spicy cornbread tastes best made with medium salsa. If you use mild, add 2 or 3 drops of hot pepper sauce. The recipe works best with butter or non-reduced-fat margarine—it's best not to try to substitute in this recipe.

1 cup yellow cornmeal

3/4 cup all-purpose or unbleached white flour

2 Tbsp sugar

2 tsp baking powder

1/8 tsp salt

2 Tbsp softened butter or regular margarine

3/4 cup low-fat (1%) milk

1 large egg white

1/3 cup medium chunky salsa

1. Preheat the oven to 400 degrees. Coat an 8-inch square baking pan with nonstick spray.
2. In a medium bowl, combine the cornmeal, flour, sugar, baking powder, and salt.
3. Cut in the butter with a pastry cutter or two forks until well combined. Add the milk, egg white, and salsa, and stir in with a few swift strokes.
4. Transfer the batter to the prepared pan, and spread it out to the edges of the pan using the back of a large spoon. Bake for 17 to 21 minutes or until the cornbread is lightly browned and a toothpick inserted in the center comes out clean.
5. Serve warm. Store leftover cornbread tightly wrapped at room temperature.

Exchanges

1 1/2 Starch

1/2 Saturated Fat

Calories 148

Total Fat 4 g

Saturated Fat 2 g

Calories from Fat 33

Cholesterol 31 mg

Sodium 180 mg

Carbohydrate 25 g

Dietary Fiber 1 g

Sugars 4 g

Protein 4 g

Preparation Time: 30 minutes

Serves 15

Serving Size: 1 piece

Exchanges

1 1/2 Starch

1/2 Monounsaturated Fat

Calories 131

Total Fat 3 g

Saturated Fat 1 g

Calories from Fat 27

Cholesterol 0 mg

Sodium 118 mg

Carbohydrate 23 g

Dietary Fiber 1 g

Sugars 2 g

Protein 3 g

Onion and Garlic Focaccia

This Italian peasant bread is easy and fun to make at home, but you do have to wait for the dough to rise. Water temperature is important for good results. If the water is too hot, it will kill the yeast. If it's too cold, the yeast won't make the dough rise. If you have a heavy-duty mixer equipped with a bread hook, use it to knead the dough; otherwise, knead by hand.

2 3/4–3 cups all-purpose white flour, divided
1 cup finely chopped onion
2 garlic cloves, minced
2 Tbsp olive oil
1 tsp Italian seasoning
1 tsp sugar
3/4–1 tsp salt
1 packet quick-acting dry yeast
1 scant cup water (125–130 degrees F)
3–4 drops hot pepper sauce
1 Tbsp olive oil
1 cup chopped onion
1 garlic clove, minced
1 tsp Italian seasoning

1. In a large mixing bowl, combine 1 1/2 cups of the flour, onion, garlic, oil, Italian seasoning, sugar, salt, and yeast. Add the warm water and hot pepper sauce. Beat with an electric mixer on low speed for 1 minute, scraping bowl frequently.

2. Increase the speed to medium, and beat 1 minute, scraping bowl frequently. Stir in enough of the remaining flour, 1/2 cup at a time, to make dough easy to handle. Form into a ball.
3. Use mixer bread hook to knead dough for 3 to 5 minutes until very cohesive, or turn out onto a lightly floured board and knead with lightly oiled hands 5 to 8 minutes until very cohesive.
4. Transfer the dough to a nonstick 9 1/2- by 13-inch pan. Press and spread dough to cover bottom surface of pan, making thickness even. Cover with nonstick spray-coated plastic wrap.
5. Allow to rise in a warm place 40 to 45 minutes, until dough has grown about 1/2 inch higher. Poke random indentation in the dough with your finger to create an uneven surface.
6. Preheat the oven to 400 degrees. Bake bread for 15 minutes. Meanwhile, in a small skillet, combine oil, onion, garlic, and Italian seasoning. Cook over medium heat, stirring frequently, until the onion is tender. Set aside.
7. Remove the bread from the oven, and spread the onion mixture evenly over the top. Return the bread to the oven, and bake an additional 15 to 20 minutes until lightly browned on top.
8. Remove the bread from the pan. Cool on a wire rack. Cut into 15 rectangles. When cooled, wrap tightly in plastic wrap. The bread will keep for 1 to 2 days at room temperature. Freeze for longer storage.

Preparation Time: 15 minutes

Serves 12

Serving Size: 1 egg roll

Baked Egg Rolls

It's fun to experiment at home with foods you've previously only eaten in restaurants. If you love egg rolls, here's a baked version that's far lower in calories than the deep-fried variety. About a cup of freshly chopped mushrooms can be substituted for part of the bean sprouts or cabbage.

1 Tbsp lite soy sauce
1 tsp cornstarch
1/2 tsp rice or white vinegar
1/4 tsp packed brown sugar
2 tsp Asian sesame oil
1/2 cup thinly sliced green onion tops
2 cups fresh bean sprouts
2 cups finely chopped Chinese cabbage
1 cup small cooked shrimp, chopped
12 egg roll wrappers
Nonstick cooking spray

1. Preheat the oven to 400 degrees. Spray a large baking sheet with nonstick spray coating and set aside. In a small bowl, mix together the soy sauce, cornstarch, and vinegar until smooth. Stir in the sugar. Set aside.
2. In a large nonstick skillet, combine the oil, onion, bean sprouts, and cabbage. Cook over medium-high heat, stirring frequently, about 3 minutes, or until the vegetables are softened. Stir in the reserved cornstarch mixture and the shrimp, and cook 1 or 2 minutes longer or until the sauce has thickened. Remove to a strainer, and drain off excess liquid.

Exchanges
1 Starch
1 Vegetable

Calories 117
Total Fat 1 g
Saturated Fat 0 g
Calories from Fat 13
Cholesterol 24 mg
Sodium 265 mg
Carbohydrate 21 g
Dietary Fiber 2 g
Sugars 1 g
Protein 6 g

3. To fill each egg roll, lay a wrapper on a flat surface with one corner facing you. Lay about 3 Tbsp of filling in a line horizontally across the center of the wrapper, leaving about 11/2 inches at each pointed end. Fold the pointed end of the wrapper facing you over the filling. Fold in the pointed ends at the sides of the wrapper over the filling.
4. Brush the remaining pointed end of the wrapper with cold water. Fold the remaining end of the wrapper over the filling, rolling to make the traditional egg roll shape. Transfer to the baking sheet. Spray the egg rolls lightly with nonstick cooking spray.
5. Bake for 13 minutes, or until the wrappers are crisped. The egg rolls are best served hot from the oven. Egg rolls can be cooled, covered, and refrigerated for up to 24 hours before serving. Rewarm in a 350-degree oven for 9 to 11 minutes.

Preparation Time:
20 minutes

Serves 17

Serving Size:
2 crackers

Herbed Crackers

Yes, you really can bake your own crackers instead of getting them out of a package. These are so flavorful that they need no topping. However, if you like, you can serve them with some cheese or a spread.

1/2 cup plus 1 Tbsp white flour
1/3 cup oat bran
1 tsp instant minced onions
1 garlic clove, minced
1/4 tsp baking soda
1/4 tsp dried thyme leaves
1/2 tsp basil
1/4 tsp salt
Pinch white pepper
1 1/2 Tbsp olive oil
1/4 cup low-fat buttermilk

1. Preheat the oven to 350 degrees. Spray a large baking sheet that is rimless on at least 2 sides with nonstick spray coating. Or use the back of a rimmed baking sheet.
2. In a medium bowl, combine the flour, oat bran, onions, garlic, baking soda, thyme, basil, salt, and pepper.
3. Stir to mix well. Add the oil and buttermilk, and stir with a large spoon until thoroughly combined. If necessary, work in the last of the flour mixture with your fingertips. Gather the dough into a ball.

Exchanges

1/2 Starch

Calories 35
Total Fat 1 g
Saturated Fat 0 g
Calories from Fat 13
Cholesterol 0 mg
Sodium 57 mg
Carbohydrate 5 g
Dietary Fiber 0 g
Sugars 1 g
Protein 1 g

4. Place the dough ball on the prepared baking sheet. Cover with wax paper, and roll the dough into a 10- by 14-inch rectangle. Try to keep the thickness of the dough as even as possible, as thick crackers will not be as crisp. Cut and patch the dough if necessary to make the sides of the rectangle straight. Gently peel off and discard the wax paper immediately after rolling out the dough.
5. Prick the dough all over with the tines of a fork. Then use a sharp knife, pizza cutter, or pastry wheel to cut the rolled-out dough into squares about 1 1/2 by 2 inches on a side, leaving the dough in place on the baking sheet.
6. Bake in the center of the oven for 12 to 15 minutes, or until the crackers on the edges of the sheet are lightly browned and crisp. Remove the baking sheet from the oven, and separate the browned crackers from the rest of the sheet with a metal spatula.
7. Transfer the browned crackers to a wire rack to cool, and return the baking sheet to the oven. Continue baking, checking the crackers about every 1 1/2 to 2 minutes and removing them from the sheet when they are done.
8. Continue until all of the crackers are lightly browned. When the crackers are slightly cooled, separate any that are still stuck together. Cool completely on a metal rack. Crackers will keep for up to a week in an air-tight container.

Crowd Pleasers

There are times when you don't want to fuss with a sit-down meal, but you do want to serve snacks that guests can enjoy. If the guys are coming over for the Super Bowl, give them Bean and Pasta Soup with Sausage, Chili Con Queso, or Black and Red Bean Tortilla Bake.

Or, for the ladies' bridge club, set out Salmon Mousse or Stuffed Artichoke Hearts. For an afternoon open house, try Cocktail Meatballs, Italian Chicken Nuggets, or Stuffed Mushrooms. Almost all of the recipes in the chapter are easily doubled if you want to feed an even larger crowd.

Notice that I've come up with a sneaky way to make better-for-you meatballs. Instead of using all ground beef, I've mixed in some ground turkey breast meat. When combined this way, the turkey takes on the flavor of the beef, and even ground turkey haters like my husband can't detect it.

The secret is in using a mixture of slightly less than half ground turkey breast. And be sure to use turkey breast, since it's far lower in fat than "lean" ground turkey, which contains high-fat dark meat and skin.

When I buy ground turkey, I use some at once and divide the rest into 4- to 6-ounce portions that I freeze for later use.

Bean and Pasta Soup with Sausage

Here's an easy but delicious bean soup that cooks quickly and can be packed in a thermos and taken to a football game or Fall tailgate picnic. You can also serve it for a quick lunch or dinner entree.

Preparation Time: 20 minutes

Serves 6

Serving Size: 3/4 cup

1 medium onion, chopped
1 large celery stalk, minced
1 garlic clove, minced
2 tsp olive oil
3 cups fat-free, low-sodium or regular chicken broth, divided
1 15-oz can cannellini beans, rinsed and well drained
1 8-oz can low-sodium or regular tomato sauce
1 tsp Italian seasoning
2–3 drops hot pepper sauce (optional)
3 oz reduced-fat beef sausage
1 oz angel hair pasta broken into 2-inch pieces (about 1/2 cup)
Salt to taste (optional)

1. In a small Dutch oven or similar pot, combine the onion, celery, garlic, oil, and 1/4 cup broth. Cook over medium heat, stirring frequently, for 6 to 7 minutes or until the onion is tender.
2. Add the remaining broth, beans, tomato sauce, Italian seasoning, and hot pepper sauce (if desired). Bring to a boil over high heat. Reduce the heat and simmer, uncovered, stirring occasionally, 15 minutes.
3. Bring the soup to a boil. Stir in the sausage and pasta. Reduce the heat and cook at a low boil 4 or 5 minutes until the pasta is tender. Add salt to taste, if desired.

Exchanges

1 Starch
1 Vegetable
1 Very Lean Meat

Calories 147
Total Fat 2 g
Saturated Fat 0 g
Calories from Fat 21
Cholesterol 6 mg
Sodium 573 mg
Carbohydrate 23 g
Dietary Fiber 4 g
Sugars 5 g
Protein 9 g

Preparation Time: 15 minutes

Serves 9

Serving Size: 1 cup

Bean and Corn Con Carne Soup

Here's another quick but hearty soup that's perfect for the football crowd. While there's only a little meat in the soup, it lends both flavor and texture.

1/2 lb reduced-fat ground beef

1 large onion, finely chopped

3 3/4 cups beef broth (2 14 1/2-oz cans)

1 14 1/2-oz can low-sodium or regular stewed tomatoes

2 15 1/2-oz cans low-sodium or regular kidney beans, rinsed and well drained

1 1/2 cups loose-pack frozen corn kernels

2 tsp chili powder, or to taste

1 tsp cumin

1/4 tsp black pepper

1/2 tsp salt or to taste (optional)

1. In a large, heavy pot, combine the ground beef and onion. Cook over medium heat, stirring frequently and breaking up the meat with a large spoon, for 5 to 6 minutes or until browned. If the meat sticks to the pot, add a small amount of the broth.
2. Add the broth, tomatoes, beans, corn, chili powder, cumin, pepper, and salt (if desired). Stir to mix well.
3. Bring the soup to a boil. Cover the pot, lower the heat, and simmer 20 to 25 minutes, stirring occasionally. With a large, shallow spoon, skim off and discard any fat from the top of the soup.
4. Serve at once, or refrigerate and rewarm. This soup keeps for 4 to 5 days in the refrigerator.

Exchanges

1 1/2 Starch

1 Vegetable

1 Very Lean Meat

Calories 167

Total Fat 2 g

Saturated Fat 0 g

Calories from Fat 16

Cholesterol 14 mg

Sodium 373 mg

Carbohydrate 26 g

Dietary Fiber 6 g

Sugars 5 g

Protein 13 g

Broccoli-Cheese Soup

Preparation Time:
15 minutes

Serves 9

Serving Size:
3/4 cup

Expand your horizons—try this simple soup when you want to feed a crowd of hungry snackers. It's delicious either hot or cold.

3 1/2 cups fat-free, low-sodium or regular chicken broth

1 cup low-fat (1%) milk

3 cups small broccoli florets

1 garlic clove, minced

1/4 tsp dry mustard

1/8 tsp ground celery seed

2–3 drops hot pepper sauce

1/4 tsp salt, or to taste (optional)

2 1/2 cups instant mashed potatoes

1 cup reduced-fat Cheddar cheese

1. In a small soup pot, combine the broth, milk, broccoli, garlic, mustard, celery seed, hot pepper sauce, and salt (if desired). Bring to a boil. Reduce the heat, cover, and simmer 5 or 6 minutes until the broccoli is tender.
2. Gradually add the mashed potatoes, stirring to prevent lumps. Break up the broccoli florets slightly with a potato masher. Simmer the soup, stirring frequently, an additional 2 or 3 minutes to combine the flavors. Turn down the heat so that the soup is not boiling. Gradually add the cheese, stirring to blend well. Serve hot.
3. Cover and refrigerate leftover soup. This soup keeps in the refrigerator 3 to 4 days. Reheat individual servings in the microwave.

Exchanges

1 Starch

1 Very Lean Meat

Calories 120

Total Fat 3 g

Saturated Fat 2 g

Calories from Fat 29

Cholesterol 10 mg

Sodium 385 mg

Carbohydrate 16 g

Dietary Fiber 2 g

Sugars 3 g

Protein 9 g

Preparation Time: 18 minutes

Serves 14

Serving Size: 2 nuggets

Italian Chicken Nuggets

These bite-sized, crispy-tender chicken pieces are especially good with a dipping sauce, such as low-fat Italian dressing, barbecue sauce, or the Mustard Sauce on page 159. To speed preparation, you can coat the chicken with the sour cream mixture in advance and refrigerate for up to 6 hours.

1/4 cup fat-free sour cream

1 tsp Italian seasoning

1/4 tsp salt, or to taste (optional)

2–3 drops hot pepper sauce

1 lb boneless, skinless chicken breast, cut into bite-sized pieces

1/2 cup Italian-style commercial bread crumbs

1. Preheat the oven to 450 degrees. Coat a large baking sheet with nonstick spray coating and set aside.
2. In a large bowl, combine the sour cream, Italian seasoning, salt (if desired), and hot pepper sauce. Stir to mix well. Stir in the chicken pieces, and stir to coat well.
3. Place the bread crumbs in a medium bowl. Roll the chicken pieces a few at a time in the bread crumbs. Set pieces on baking sheet. Bake in preheated oven 7 to 9 minutes or until the chicken is cooked through but still moist. Serve warm with toothpicks.
4. Cover and refrigerate leftovers, which will keep 1 to 2 days in the refrigerator.

Exchanges

1 Lean Meat

Calories 58

Total Fat 1 g

Saturated Fat 0 g

Calories from Fat 8

Cholesterol 20 mg

Sodium 139 mg

Carbohydrate 4 g

Dietary Fiber 0 g

Sugars 1 g

Protein 8 g

Chili Con Queso Dip

Preparation Time:
18 minutes

Serves 32

Serving Size:
2 Tbsp and
4 chips

Here's a crowd pleaser you'll serve frequently.

5 oz lean ground beef
4 oz ground turkey breast
2 cups frozen mixed pepper and onion stir-fry
1 garlic clove, minced
1 16-oz jar mild salsa
1 8-oz can low-sodium or regular tomato sauce
2 Tbsp tomato paste
1 tsp chili powder
1 tsp cumin
1/2 tsp salt, or to taste (optional)
1 cup grated reduced-fat Cheddar cheese
4 fat-free tortilla chips per person

1. In a small Dutch oven or large pot, combine the ground beef, ground turkey, pepper and onion mixture, and garlic. Cook over medium heat until the beef is brown, breaking up any large pieces of onion, about 5 to 6 minutes.
2. Add the salsa, tomato sauce, tomato paste, chili powder, cumin, and salt (if desired). Stir to mix well. Cover and simmer 15 minutes, stirring frequently, to allow the flavors to blend. Remove from the heat. Stir in the cheese until melted.
3. Serve warm in a chafing dish or on a hot plate. Serve with fat-free tortilla chips. Cover and refrigerate leftovers. Leftovers keep for 3 to 4 days in the refrigerator.

Exchanges

1/2 Starch

Calories 47
Total Fat 1 g
Saturated Fat 1 g
Calories from Fat 10
Cholesterol 7 mg
Sodium 97 mg
Carbohydrate 6 g
Dietary Fiber 1 g
Sugars 1 g
Protein 4 g

Preparation Time:
45 minutes

Serves 34

Serving Size:
2 meatballs

Exchanges

1 Very Lean Meat

Calories 36
Total Fat 1 g
Saturated Fat 0 g
Calories from Fat 5
Cholesterol 12 mg
Sodium 11 mg
Carbohydrate 3 g
Dietary Fiber 0 g
Sugars 1 g
Protein 5 g

Cocktail Meatballs

These wonderful meatballs taste like they're all beef, but they're a lot healthier because they contain fresh ground turkey breast. Mixed with lean ground beef, the turkey takes on a beefy flavor and is virtually undetectable. Don't substitute ordinary ground turkey, as it contains fatty dark meat and sometimes skin.

Meatballs:

1 lb reduced-fat ground beef
9 oz fresh ground turkey breast
1/2 cup quick-cooking rolled oats
1 medium onion, finely chopped
1 garlic clove, minced
1 tsp dried thyme leaves
1 tsp dried marjoram leaves
1 large egg white
1/2 tsp salt (optional)
1/8 tsp black pepper

Sauce:

1 15-oz can low-sodium or regular tomato sauce
1/2 cup water
2 Tbsp packed brown sugar
1 Tbsp balsamic vinegar
1 garlic clove, minced
3/4 tsp dry mustard
2–3 drops hot pepper sauce
1/4 tsp allspice

1. Preheat the oven to 400 degrees. Spray the bottom and sides of a large baking pan with nonstick spray coating. Set aside.
2. In a large bowl, combine the ground beef, ground turkey, oats, onion, garlic, thyme, marjoram, egg white, salt (if desired), and pepper. Mix well. Roll into 68 1-inch balls.
3. Place the balls on the baking pan. Bake for 10 to 13 minutes, or until the meatballs are browned on all sides, turning once during browning.
4. Meanwhile, in a Dutch oven or similar heavy pot, mix together the tomato sauce, water, brown sugar, vinegar, garlic, mustard, hot pepper sauce, and allspice.
5. When the meatballs are browned, transfer them to the sauce with a large slotted spoon, cover, and bring to a boil. Reduce the heat and simmer 30 to 35 minutes, stirring occasionally and being careful not to break up the balls. Skim any fat from the surface of the liquid.
6. Serve immediately, or cover and refrigerate. Meatballs can be refrigerated 2 to 3 days before serving or frozen for up to a month.

Preparation Time: 35 minutes

Serves 21

Serving Size: 2 meatballs

Exchanges

1/2 Fruit

1 Very Lean Meat

Calories 56

Total Fat 1 g

Saturated Fat 0 g

Calories from Fat 7

Cholesterol 18 mg

Sodium 71 mg

Carbohydrate 4 g

Dietary Fiber 0 g

Sugars 4 g

Protein 8 g

Hawaiian Meatballs

The surprise ingredient in these tasty meatballs is pumpkin pie spice! Like the meatballs in the previous recipe, they combine ground turkey breast with lean ground beef, although the addition of the turkey is undetectable in the finished meatballs.

Meatballs:

1 lb reduced-fat ground beef

8 oz ground turkey breast

1 small onion, finely chopped

2 garlic cloves, minced

1/4 cup quick-cooking rolled oats

1 large egg white

1 tsp pumpkin pie spice

1 tsp dried thyme leaves

1/4 tsp salt, or to taste (optional)

Pinch black pepper

Sauce:

1 1/2 cups orange juice

1 8-oz can crushed pineapple

2 Tbsp lite soy sauce

1/2 Tbsp packed light brown sugar

1/2 tsp ginger

1/8 tsp salt (optional)

1. Preheat the oven to 375 degrees. In a large bowl, combine the ground beef, ground turkey, onion, garlic, oats, egg white, pumpkin pie spice, thyme, salt (if desired), and pepper. Mix well.

2. Roll the meat mixture into about 42 balls, and arrange in a large nonstick spray-coated baking pan. Bake in the upper half of the oven for 12 to 15 minutes or until browned, turning once during browning.
3. Meanwhile, combine the orange juice, pineapple, soy sauce, brown sugar, ginger, and salt (if desired), in a 3-quart flame-proof casserole. Heat the ingredients to a simmer.
4. With a large slotted spoon, transfer the meatballs to the sauce mixture, and simmer uncovered, stirring occasionally. Continue simmering for about 30 to 35 minutes, until the sauce has cooked down and thickened so that it coats the meatballs.
5. Serve at once, or cover and refrigerate. Meatballs will keep in the refrigerator for 3 to 4 days.

Preparation Time: 15 minutes

Serves 10

Serving Size: 3 pieces

Middle Eastern-Style Chicken

Serve these spicy chicken bits in a casserole on a hot tray or in a chafing dish. For a buffet variation, you can serve the chicken and sauce over couscous.

1 lb boneless, skinless chicken breast, trimmed of all fat and cut into bite-sized pieces
2 cups frozen mixed pepper and onion stir-fry
2 garlic cloves, minced
2 tsp olive oil
1 cup fat-free, low-sodium or regular chicken broth
1 14 1/2-oz can low-sodium or regular diced tomato
1/2 cup dark raisins
1 large bay leaf
1 1/2 tsp dried thyme leaves
1 tsp cumin
1/4 tsp allspice
1/8 tsp cloves
1/8 tsp black pepper
Salt to taste (optional)

1. In a nonstick skillet coated with nonstick spray coating, cook the chicken pieces over medium heat, turning frequently, until they begin to brown.
2. Add the onion and pepper mixture, garlic, oil, and 1 Tbsp of the broth to the skillet. Stir up any browned bits from the bottom of the pan. Raise the heat and bring to a boil.

Exchanges

1/2 Carbohydrate

1 Lean Meat

Calories 99
Total Fat 2 g
Saturated Fat 0 g
Calories from Fat 20
Cholesterol 27 mg
Sodium 106 mg
Carbohydrate 9 g
Dietary Fiber 1 g
Sugars 7 g
Protein 11 g

3. Lower heat again and cook over medium heat, stirring frequently, 2 or 3 minutes, or until the onion is slightly softened. Add the remaining broth, tomato, raisins, bay leaf, thyme, cumin, allspice, cloves, and black pepper.
4. Bring to a boil, reduce the heat, and simmer, uncovered, about 20 minutes, or until the chicken is tender and the sauce has cooked down slightly. Remove the bay leaf and discard. Add salt to taste (if desired).
5. Serve at once, or transfer to a casserole, cover, and refrigerate. The chicken will keep for 2 to 3 days in the refrigerator.

Preparation Time: 15 minutes

Serves 12

Serving Size: 1 piece

Exchanges

1 1/2 Starch

1 Vegetable

1 Medium Fat Meat

Calories 228

Total Fat 6 g

Saturated Fat 3 g

Calories from Fat 55

Cholesterol 15 mg

Sodium 411 mg

Carbohydrate 30 g

Dietary Fiber 6 g

Sugars 5 g

Protein 15 g

Black and Red Bean Tortilla Bake

Tex-Mex flavors predominate in this easy layered bake. It's great as part of a buffet or when you want to feed a gang of hungry male snackers.

Bake:

2 cups frozen mixed pepper and onion stir-fry

2 garlic cloves, minced

2 tsp olive oil

1 cup mild salsa

1 15-oz can low-sodium or regular tomato sauce

1 1/2 tsp cumin

1 tsp chili powder

1 15-oz can black beans, rinsed and well drained

1 16-oz can low-sodium or regular kidney beans, rinsed and well drained

12–14 6-inch corn tortillas

1 cup low-fat (1%) cottage cheese

2 cups shredded reduced-fat Cheddar cheese, divided

Garnish:

1 large tomato, chopped

1/4 cup thinly sliced green onion tops

1/2 cup fat-free or reduced-fat sour cream

1. Preheat the oven to 350 degrees. In a small pot or very large saucepan, combine the pepper-onion mixture, garlic, and oil. Cook over medium heat, stirring frequently, until the onion is soft, about 5 or 6 minutes.

2. Add the salsa, tomato sauce, cumin, and chili powder. Simmer, uncovered, for 5 minutes. Stir in the black beans and kidney beans. Remove from the burner.
3. Spread one half of the bean mixture evenly in the bottom of a 9 1/2- by 13-inch baking pan. Top with one half of the tortillas in an overlapping layer. With the back of a large spoon, spread the cottage cheese evenly over the tortillas.
4. Top with one half of the Cheddar cheese. Add the remaining tortillas, then the remaining bean mixture. Cover with aluminum foil and bake for 30 to 35 minutes or until heated through.
5. Sprinkle with the remaining Cheddar cheese, and bake uncovered an additional 5 to 6 minutes or until the cheese is partially melted. To serve, cut into 12 rectangles, and garnish with tomatoes, green onion, and sour cream.

Preparation Time: 20 minutes

Serves 12

Serving Size: 1 piece

Spanakopita Bake

Frozen phyllo dough works well for creating a variety of pastries. Here I've used it in a Greek-style spinach and cheese casserole. Be sure to allow 5 hours to thaw frozen phyllo at room temperature. If you forget to thaw the dough, you can do it in the microwave. However, sheets of microwave-thawed dough may stick together in some places, making them harder to work with.

Incidentally, while phyllo itself has no fat, restaurant phyllo dishes are likely to be high in fat, since the dough is liberally slathered with butter. In my recipes, the fat content is held to a minimum by substituting nonstick spray coating and using butter very sparingly.

Exchanges

1 Starch

1 Medium Fat Meat

1/2 Saturated Fat

Calories 177

Total Fat 8 g

Saturated Fat 4 g

Calories from Fat 72

Cholesterol 40 mg

Sodium 476 mg

Carbohydrate 14 g

Dietary Fiber 2 g

Sugars 3 g

Protein 12 g

1 1/2 Tbsp olive oil
1 large onion, chopped
1 1-lb bag cut-leaf, loose-pack frozen spinach
2 1/2 tsp dried dill weed
1/4 tsp salt (optional)
1/4 tsp black pepper
6 oz crumbled feta cheese
3 cups low-fat cottage cheese (1% fat)
2 large egg whites plus 1 yolk, beaten together
7 large phyllo sheets, thawed
2 Tbsp melted butter
Butter-flavored nonstick spray coating

1. Spray a 9- by 13 1/2-inch baking pan with the nonstick spray coating and set aside. Preheat the oven to 375 degrees.

2. In a nonstick skillet over medium heat, combine the oil and onion. Cook the onion, stirring frequently, until it is soft but not browned. Stir in the spinach. Cover and cook gently for 4 to 5 minutes, stirring occasionally, and breaking up any large lumps of spinach if necessary.
3. Remove the skillet from the burner. Stir in the dill, salt (if desired), pepper, and cheeses. Stir in the eggs.
4. Unwrap the phyllo onto wax paper. Cover with additional wax paper and a barely damp tea towel. Working quickly, lay a phyllo layer in the bottom of the pan. Spray with the butter-flavored nonstick spray coating. Add three more layers, spraying each.
5. Cover with the filling, spreading the mixture evenly with the back of a spoon. Top with 3 phyllo sheets, brushing each layer lightly with the melted butter.
6. Bake for about 35 to 37 minutes or until the filling is cooked through and the top layer of phyllo begins to brown. Serve at once, or cover and refrigerate up to 24 hours before serving. Warm in a 350-degree oven for about 20 minutes.

Salmon Mousse

Preparation Time: 25 minutes

Serves 16

Serving Size: 2 Tbsp

This salmon mousse looks very elegant when served in a fish mold. And the flavor is wonderful. Serve it with fat-free crackers or thinly sliced French bread. If you use a fish mold with a rounded bottom, check ahead of time to see that the mold will remain upright when the mousse is poured in. If not, make a supporting nest of crumpled aluminum foil.

1 15-oz can red salmon, drained
1 envelope unflavored gelatin
1/4 cup cold water
1/3 cup boiling water
1/4 cup reduced-fat mayonnaise
1/4 cup reduced-fat Neufchâtel cheese, at room temperature, cut into 3 or 4 pieces
3 Tbsp thinly sliced green onion tops
2 Tbsp lemon juice
2 3/4 tsp fresh dill leaves or 1 tsp dried dill weed
2 tsp prepared white horseradish
1/4 tsp salt, or to taste (optional)
3–4 drops hot pepper sauce
1/4 cup finely chopped fresh parsley

1. Remove the skin and bones from the salmon. Break the salmon meat into small pieces. Set aside in a medium bowl.
2. In a small bowl, sprinkle the gelatin over the cold water. Let stand 5 minutes to soften. Add the boiling water and stir to dissolve.

Exchanges

1 Lean Meat

Calories 53
Total Fat 3 g
Saturated Fat 1 g
Calories from Fat 28
Cholesterol 16 mg
Sodium 156 mg
Carbohydrate 1 g
Dietary Fiber 0 g
Sugars 0 g
Protein 5 g

3. In a food processor container, combine the salmon, mayonnaise, Neufchâtel, onion, lemon juice, dill, horseradish, salt (if desired), hot pepper sauce, and gelatin mixture. Process until almost completely smooth. Stir in the parsley.
4. Pour into a nonstick spray-coated 2- to 3-cup fish mold or other mold. Cover with plastic wrap, and chill until firm, at least 4 hours or overnight. If the fish mold is unstable, lay on a plate and support with crumpled aluminum foil to keep the mold upright.
5. To unmold, run a thin knife around the edge of the mold. Dip the top of the mold in a pan of hot water for just a few seconds. Wipe dry and cover the mold with a serving platter. Invert. If necessary, shake to loosen mold.
6. Garnish with parsley or watercress. Serve with nonfat crackers. The leftover salmon mousse can be covered and refrigerated for 3 to 4 days.

Preparation Time:
15 minutes

Serves 28

Serving Size:
2 Tbsp

Mexican Layered Spread

This full-flavored Mexican spread is a big hit at parties. Serve the spread with fat-free tortilla chips or toasted whole-wheat pita triangles.

1 16-oz can fat-free refried beans

1 cup fat-free sour cream

1 cup mild chunky salsa

1 cup shredded reduced-fat Cheddar cheese

1–3 Tbsp thinly sliced green onion tops

1. Place the beans in a 9-inch pie plate, spreading them out evenly with the back of a serving spoon. Spread the sour cream evenly over the beans.
2. Spread the salsa evenly over the sour cream. Sprinkle evenly with the cheese. Top with the sliced green onion.
3. Serve at once, or cover and refrigerate 2 to 3 hours or up to 24 hours before serving. The spread will keep for 3 to 4 days in the refrigerator.

Exchanges

1/2 Starch

Calories 37

Total Fat 1 g

Saturated Fat 1 g

Calories from Fat 8

Cholesterol 3 mg

Sodium 138 mg

Carbohydrate 4 g

Dietary Fiber 1 g

Sugars 1 g

Protein 3 g

Stuffed Artichoke Hearts

Preparation Time: 15 minutes

Serves 8

Serving Size: 1 heart

Here's the kind of recipe I like: delicious, quick, easy, and elegant. The recipe is simple to double if you want to make a larger batch.

1/3 cup chopped ripe tomato

2 Tbsp chopped chives or sliced green onion tops

1 Tbsp grated Parmesan cheese

1 tsp olive oil

Dash salt, or to taste (optional)

2 drops hot pepper sauce (optional)

1 14-oz can whole artichoke hearts, well drained

1. In a small bowl, mix together the tomato, chives, Parmesan cheese, oil, and salt (if desired).
2. Remove coarse outer leaves from the artichokes. Cut a small sliver from the bottom of the hearts so they will stand upright. Set the artichoke hearts, bottom side down, on a plate.
3. Carefully open the leaves to form a cavity. Spoon the stuffing into the cavity in the hearts, dividing evenly.
4. Serve at once or cover and refrigerate several hours or overnight before serving.

Exchanges

1 Vegetable

Calories 22

Total Fat 1 g

Saturated Fat 0 g

Calories from Fat 9

Cholesterol 1 mg

Sodium 104 mg

Carbohydrate 3 g

Dietary Fiber 1 g

Sugars 1 g

Protein 1 g

Preparation Time: 25 minutes

Serves 8

Serving Size: 2 potato halves

Feta-Stuffed New Potatoes

If you like the taste of feta cheese, you'll love these tiny, stuffed potato snacks.

8 new brown- or red-skinned potatoes no larger than 1 1/2 inches in diameter, scrubbed but not peeled

1/4 cup crumbled feta cheese

1/4 cup fat-free sour cream

1 Tbsp reduced-fat mayonnaise

1 large celery stalk, finely chopped

1 Tbsp chopped chives

1. In a steamer, steam the potatoes 17 to 19 minutes, or until just barely tender. Meanwhile, while potatoes are cooking, in a small bowl combine the feta, sour cream, mayonnaise, celery, and chives. Stir to mix well. Set aside.
2. When the potatoes are tender, cool slightly under cold running water. Cut the potatoes in half. Cut a small slice off the rounded part of each half so that the half will stand upright. With a melon baller or small spoon, hollow out the center of each potato half, leaving a 1/4-inch-thick wall. (Reserve the potato centers for another use, if desired.)
3. Fill the potatoes with the cheese mixture and serve. Or cover and refrigerate up to 24 hours before serving. The stuffed potatoes will keep in the refrigerator 2 to 3 days.

Exchanges

1/2 Starch

1/2 Fat

Calories 58

Total Fat 1 g

Saturated Fat 1 g

Calories from Fat 12

Cholesterol 4 mg

Sodium 76 mg

Carbohydrate 9 g

Dietary Fiber 1 g

Sugars 2 g

Protein 2 g

Stuffed Mushrooms

Preparation Time: 15 minutes

Serves 10

Serving Size: 1 mushroom

Always a hit, these stuffed mushrooms are a snap to prepare. If you wash them, be sure to dry them thoroughly before stuffing them.

1 lb large white mushrooms (about 10–12), cleaned and well dried with paper towels

2 Tbsp chopped chives or thinly sliced green onion tops

2 Tbsp reduced-fat mayonnaise

3 Tbsp fat-free sour cream

2 Tbsp grated Parmesan cheese

5 Tbsp Italian seasoned bread crumbs

1 Tbsp balsamic vinegar

2–3 drops hot pepper sauce (optional)

1. Preheat the broiler. Spray a baking sheet with nonstick spray. Trim the mushroom stems. Pull out the stems, chop, and reserve. Lay the mushrooms, rounded side down, on the baking sheet.
2. In a small bowl, combine 1/3 cup of the mushroom stems, chives, mayonnaise, sour cream, cheese, bread crumbs, vinegar, and hot pepper sauce (if desired). Stir to mix well.
3. Stuff each mushroom with the cheese mixture. Broil 2 inches from the broiler until the stuffing begins to brown, about 2 to 4 minutes. Serve warm.

Exchanges

1 Vegetable

1/2 Fat

Calories 41

Total Fat 2 g

Saturated Fat 1 g

Calories from Fat 14

Cholesterol 3 mg

Sodium 159 mg

Carbohydrate 5 g

Dietary Fiber 0 g

Sugars 1 g

Protein 2 g

Preparation Time:
8 minutes

Serves 18

Serving Size:
2 Tbsp

Shrimp Remoulade

These shrimp in spicy sauce make an elegant appetizer. Serve them on fat-free crackers or thin slices of French bread.

1/2 cup chili sauce

1/4 cup fat-free sour cream

2 Tbsp reduced-fat mayonnaise

1 garlic clove, minced

1 tsp prepared white horseradish

1 lb medium cooked shrimp, shelled and deveined

1. In a medium bowl, whisk together the chili sauce, sour cream, mayonnaise, garlic, and horseradish.
2. Stir in the shrimp. Serve immediately, or cover and refrigerate several hours before serving.

Exchanges

1 Very Lean Meat

Calories 41

Total Fat 1 g

Saturated Fat 0 g

Calories from Fat 7

Cholesterol 50 mg

Sodium 162 mg

Carbohydrate 2 g

Dietary Fiber 0 g

Sugars 1 g

Protein 6 g

Vegetable Delights

This chapter answers the question, "Can vegetables be snacks?" Of course! Not only are they tasty, but they're the perfect health-conscious alternative to less nutritious treats. Try the Roasted Asparagus, Pan-Grilled Italian Vegetables, or Luscious Limas, and I'm sure you'll agree. All of these recipes are low in fat and calories and high in fiber. And the Portobello Mushroom Slices are heavenly—good enough to serve at the fanciest party.

Preparation Time:
2 minutes

Serves 1

Portobello Mushroom Slices

These portobello mushrooms—pan-grilled and tossed with a little balsamic vinegar and Parmesan cheese—are great with fresh French bread!

3 oz portobello mushroom slices (about 8 large slices)

1 tsp olive oil

Pinch salt (optional)

1/8 tsp black pepper

1 tsp balsamic vinegar

1 tsp grated Parmesan cheese

1. Spray a medium nonstick skillet with nonstick spray coating. Add the mushrooms to the skillet and brush with the oil, using a brush or your finger. Sprinkle with salt (if desired) and pepper.
2. Cook over medium to medium-high heat 6 to 7 minutes or until the mushrooms have exuded their juices, softened, and begun to brown.
3. Remove the pan from the heat. Stir in the vinegar and cheese and toss to coat the mushrooms. Serve at once.

Exchanges

1 Vegetable

1 Monounsaturated Fat

Calories 72

Total Fat 6 g

Saturated Fat 2 g

Calories from Fat 50

Cholesterol 3 mg

Sodium 46 mg

Carbohydrate 4 g

Dietary Fiber 1 g

Sugars 2 g

Protein 3 g

Florentine Potato Pancakes

Preparation Time:
6 minutes

Serves 4

Serving Size:
1 pancake

These potato pancakes get a quick start because the potatoes are first microwaved. You could omit the olive oil from the recipe if you wanted to. However, the pancakes will brown better with the oil.

2 medium red-skinned potatoes, scrubbed

1/4 cup fat-free milk

1/4 cup loose-leaf, dry-pack frozen spinach

1/2 tsp instant minced onion

Dash garlic powder

1/4 tsp salt, or to taste (optional)

1/8 tsp black pepper, or to taste

1 tsp olive oil

1/2 Tbsp grated Parmesan cheese

1. Pierce the potatoes with a fork and microwave 7 to 8 minutes on high power, turning once, until cooked through.
2. Cut the potatoes into large chunks, and transfer them to a medium bowl. Mash with a potato masher or fork. Stir in the milk, spinach, onion, garlic, salt (if desired), and pepper. Stir to mix well. Shape mixture into 4 pancakes.
3. Coat a large nonstick skillet with the oil. Cook the pancakes over medium-high heat, until browned on one side, about 2 to 3 minutes. Turn with a spatula, and brown the other side.
4. Transfer the pancakes to plates, and sprinkle with the Parmesan cheese, dividing it evenly. Serve hot. The pancakes will keep for 2 to 3 days in the refrigerator.

Exchanges

1 Starch

Calories 85

Total Fat 1 g

Saturated Fat 0 g

Calories from Fat 13

Cholesterol 1 mg

Sodium 40 mg

Carbohydrate 15 g

Dietary Fiber 2 g

Sugars 2 g

Protein 3 g

Roasted Asparagus

Preparation Time:
5 minutes

Serves 2

Serving Size:
5 spears and 1 oz bread

Once you try roasted asparagus, you'll never want to cook it any other way. This easy but elegant recipe makes a delicious snack as well as a great buffet table entree. And it's a wonderful way to include vegetables in your meal plan.

10 medium asparagus spears, well washed and coarse ends snapped off

1 tsp olive oil

1/8 tsp salt (optional)

1/2 Tbsp grated Parmesan cheese

2 thin slices toasted Italian bread

1. Preheat the oven to 400 degrees. Dry the asparagus on paper towels. Place the spears in a shallow roasting pan. Drizzle the spears with oil and turn to coat. Sprinkle on salt (if desired).
2. Roast for 10 minutes or until the spears are tender. Remove to a plate and sprinkle with Parmesan cheese. Serve on toasted Italian bread slices.

Exchanges

1 Starch

1 Vegetable

1/2 Monounsaturated Fat

Calories 120

Total Fat 4 g

Saturated Fat 1 g

Calories from Fat 37

Cholesterol 2 mg

Sodium 192 mg

Carbohydrate 17 g

Dietary Fiber 2 g

Sugars 2 g

Protein 5 g

Easy Cheese Sauce

Preparation Time:
7 minutes

Serves 8

Serving Size:
1/4 cup

Cheese sauce is a wonderful way to dress up cooked vegetables, but it can be high in fat and calories. Here's a light yet flavorful version you can make in a hurry.

1 1/2 Tbsp all-purpose or unbleached white flour
1/2 tsp dry mustard
1/2 tsp salt, or to taste (optional)
Pinch ground celery seed
2 cups reduced-fat (2%) milk
3–4 drops hot pepper sauce
1 cup grated reduced-fat Cheddar cheese

1. In a small saucepan, stir together the flour, mustard, salt (if desired), and celery seed. Slowly add the milk, stirring with a wire whisk to keep the mixture from lumping. Whisk until the flour is completely incorporated. Add the hot pepper sauce.
2. Over medium heat, cook the milk and flour mixture, whisking, until the mixture thickens, about 3 or 4 minutes. Gradually add the cheese, continuing to whisk until the cheese is completely melted.
3. Serve over vegetables, such as cooked broccoli, cauliflower, or zucchini.

Exchanges

1 Medium Fat Meat

Calories 81
Total Fat 4 g
Saturated Fat 3 g
Calories from Fat 38
Cholesterol 15 mg
Sodium 145 mg
Carbohydrate 4 g
Dietary Fiber 0 g
Sugars 3 g
Protein 7 g

Preparation Time: 12 minutes

Serves 10

Serving Size: 1/2 cup

Exchanges

1 Starch

Calories 84

Total Fat 2 g

Saturated Fat 0 g

Calories from Fat 19

Cholesterol 0 mg

Sodium 25 mg

Carbohydrate 15 g

Dietary Fiber 2 g

Sugars 5 g

Protein 2 g

Roasted Winter Vegetables

Truly delicious, roasted winter vegetables are a great way to add variety to your snacking experience. If you've enjoyed them at a trendy cafe, you'll be glad to know they're a snap to make. Starting the vegetables in the microwave shortens the cooking time considerably.

3 medium onions, cut into large chunks and separated into slices

3 cups red-skinned potatoes, cut into 1-inch pieces

1 1/2 cups baby carrots, cut in half crosswise if the carrots are large

1 medium turnip, peeled and diced

2 Tbsp water

1 1/2 Tbsp olive oil

1 garlic clove, minced

1 tsp Italian seasoning

1/2 tsp salt, or to taste (optional)

1/8 tsp black pepper

1. Preheat the oven to 450 degrees. Combine the onions, potatoes, carrots, and turnip in a medium bowl. Add the water.
2. Cover with wax paper and microwave on high power 6 to 8 minutes, stopping and stirring once, or until the vegetables are partially cooked. Drain the vegetables in a colander.
3. Transfer the vegetables to a large nonstick spray-coated baking pan or rimmed baking sheet. Drizzle with the oil. Sprinkle with the garlic, Italian seasoning, salt (if desired), and pepper. Stir to mix well.

4. Bake 30 to 40 minutes, stirring occasionally, or until the vegetables begin to brown and are tender. Serve immediately. Leftover vegetables can be covered and refrigerated for 2 to 3 days and reheated in the microwave.

Preparation Time: 10 minutes

Serves 2

Serving Size: 1/2 cup

Exchanges

1 Vegetable

1/2 Monounsaturated Fat

Calories 49

Total Fat 2 g

Saturated Fat 1 g

Calories from Fat 21

Cholesterol 0 mg

Sodium 3 mg

Carbohydrate 7 g

Dietary Fiber 1 g

Sugars 4 g

Protein 1 g

Pan-Grilled Italian Vegetables

Pan-grilled vegetables make an easy, tasty snack. If you like, substitute chopped cauliflower or broccoli for the zucchini.

1 small onion, coarsely chopped
1 garlic clove, minced
1/4 cup red or green bell pepper
1/4 cup chopped zucchini
1 tsp extra virgin olive oil
1/4 tsp Italian seasoning
Salt (optional) and pepper to taste

1. In a small nonstick skillet, combine the onion, garlic, red or green pepper, zucchini, and oil. Cook, stirring frequently, over medium heat, until the vegetables are softened and begin to brown slightly.
2. Stir in the Italian seasoning, salt (if desired), and pepper. Serve hot on a 1/2-inch slice of toasted Italian bread or on a small whole-wheat pita bread half.

Israeli Chickpeas

Preparation Time: 3 minutes

Serves 4

Serving Size: 1/2 cup

I've loved chickpeas (garbanzo beans) right from the can since I was a kid, so I was delighted to discover this quick method for making them even better.

1 15-oz can chickpeas (garbanzo beans), rinsed and well-drained

1/2 tsp seasoned salt or to taste (optional), or non-sodium seasoning

Dash black pepper, or to taste

1. Spray a large, heavy nonstick skillet with nonstick spray coating.
2. Add the chickpeas, and season with salt and pepper as desired. Cook over medium heat, shaking skillet often, until the chickpeas are lightly browned, 2 to 4 minutes.
3. Cool slightly before serving. Leftover chickpeas will keep in the refrigerator for 2 to 3 days and can be reheated in the microwave or served cold.

Exchanges

1 Starch

1 Very Lean Meat

Calories 118

Total Fat 2 g

Saturated Fat 0 g

Calories from Fat 17

Cholesterol 0 mg

Sodium 105 mg

Carbohydrate 20 g

Dietary Fiber 6 g

Sugars 3 g

Protein 6 g

Preparation Time:
15 minutes

Serves 12

Serving Size:
1/4 cup

Lentils with Cumin and Lemon

I never met a legume I didn't like, but lentils are one of my favorites. Here's an interesting way to flavor them. Because they're cooked al dente, they still have a bit of crunch. If you prefer, you can cook them to a softer consistency.

1 cup dried brown lentils, washed and sorted
1 small onion, chopped
1 garlic clove, minced
1 celery stalk, minced
2 tsp lemon juice
1 tsp cumin
1/2 tsp salt, or to taste (optional)
1/8 tsp black pepper

1. In a large saucepan, combine the lentils and 3 cups of water. Cover and bring to a boil. Reduce the heat, and simmer 18 to 20 minutes or until the lentils are tender-crisp. Drain in a colander.
2. In a medium bowl, combine the lentils, onion, garlic, celery, lemon juice, cumin, salt (if desired), and pepper. Stir to mix well.
3. Serve warm, either plain or on fat-free crackers or toasted whole-wheat bread. Or cover and refrigerate until chilled. Lentils will keep in the refrigerator for 3 to 4 days.

Exchanges

1/2 Starch

Calories 54
Total Fat 0 g
Saturated Fat 0 g
Calories from Fat 2
Cholesterol 0 mg
Sodium 4 mg
Carbohydrate 10 g
Dietary Fiber 4 g
Sugars 1 g
Protein 4 g

Luscious Limas

Preparation Time: 3 minutes

Serves 4

Serving Size: 1/2 cup

Like broccoli, lima beans inspire a strong reaction. If you like them, you'll love this recipe.

1 10-oz package frozen baby lima beans

1 cup frozen mixed pepper and onion stir-fry

2 Tbsp grated Parmesan cheese

1 tsp olive oil

1/8 tsp salt (optional)

Dash black pepper

1. In a medium saucepan over high heat, combine the lima beans, vegetables, and 3/4 cup boiling water. Return to a boil. Cover, lower the heat, and simmer 12 to 14 minutes or until the beans are tender. Drain in a colander.
2. Transfer the bean mixture to a medium bowl. Stir in the cheese, oil, salt (if desired), and pepper. Serve at once.
3. The beans will keep in the refrigerator for 3 to 4 days.

Exchanges

1/2 Starch

1/2 Fat

Calories 70

Total Fat 2 g

Saturated Fat 1 g

Calories from Fat 22

Cholesterol 4 mg

Sodium 88 mg

Carbohydrate 9 g

Dietary Fiber 3 g

Sugars 2 g

Protein 4 g

Preparation Time: 10 minutes

Serves 6

Serving Size: 3 sticks

Crispy Eggplant Sticks with Dipping Sauce

These crispy, oven-baked sticks make an unusual and very tasty snack, especially if you like the flavors of Asian cuisines.

Eggplant sticks:

1/3 cup cornmeal

1/3 cup sesame seeds

1/8 tsp each salt and black pepper

1 medium (about 1 lb) eggplant, peeled and cut into 3- by 1-inch sticks

1/3 cup liquid egg substitute

1 Tbsp lite soy sauce

Dipping sauce:

1 small garlic clove, peeled and chopped

1 1/2 tsp peeled and finely minced fresh ginger root

1 1/2 Tbsp lite soy sauce

1 1/2 Tbsp rice vinegar

1 1/2 Tbsp white wine

1 1/2 tsp packed light brown sugar, or to taste

2–4 dashes hot chili oil (optional)

1. Preheat the oven to 475 degrees. Line a 12- by 18-inch or similar large baking sheet with aluminum foil. Lightly spray with nonstick spray coating and set aside.
2. In a large shallow bowl, stir together the cornmeal, sesame seeds, salt, and pepper until well mixed. In another bowl, stir together the egg substitute and soy sauce.

Exchanges

1 Starch

1/2 Fat

Calories 109

Total Fat 4 g

Saturated Fat 1 g

Calories from Fat 38

Cholesterol 0 mg

Sodium 326 mg

Carbohydrate 14 g

Dietary Fiber 3 g

Sugars 5 g

Protein 4 g

3. In batches, dip the eggplant sticks into the egg mixture, removing with a slotted spoon and shaking off any excess. Then toss the eggplant sticks into the cornmeal mixture until evenly coated all over. Lay the sticks, separated, on the baking sheet.
4. Bake in the upper third of the oven until the sticks are nicely browned, about 8 to 10 minutes. Turn over using a spatula.
5. Return to the oven; bake sticks 6 to 8 minutes longer, or until well browned and just tender when pierced with a fork. Remove from the oven, and set aside.
6. Meanwhile, prepare the dipping sauce by stirring together the garlic, ginger, soy sauce, vinegar, wine, sugar, and chili oil (if desired).
7. Serve warm eggplant sticks with a bowl of dipping sauce on the side. The eggplant and sauce may be covered and kept in the refrigerator for 3 to 4 days. Reheat the eggplant until hot in a 400-degree oven before serving.

Preparation Time: 10 minutes

Serves 5

Serving Size: 1/2 cup

Marinated Artichoke Hearts and Cherry Tomatoes

Artichoke hearts and cherry tomatoes compliment each other very well. If you like, double this recipe and serve it to a crowd.

2 Tbsp fat-free, low-sodium or regular chicken broth

2 Tbsp olive oil (preferably extra-virgin)

2 Tbsp thinly sliced green onion tops

1 tsp lemon juice

1 tsp apple cider vinegar

1/2 tsp dried thyme leaves

1/2 tsp basil

1/8 tsp salt, or to taste (optional)

1 15-oz can artichoke heart quarters, well drained

1 cup halved cherry tomatoes (15–25, depending on size)

1. In a medium bowl, combine the broth, oil, green onion, lemon juice, vinegar, thyme, basil, and salt (if desired). Stir to mix well.
2. Remove any coarse outer leaves from the artichoke hearts. Stir the artichoke hearts and the tomatoes into the dressing, and gently toss to coat.
3. Serve at once, or cover and refrigerate up to 24 hours. Marinated vegetables will keep in the refrigerator for 3 to 4 days.

Exchanges

1 Vegetable

1 Monounsaturated Fat

Calories 74

Total Fat 6 g

Saturated Fat 1 g

Calories from Fat 52

Cholesterol 0 mg

Sodium 158 mg

Carbohydrate 5 g

Dietary Fiber 2 g

Sugars 3 g

Protein 2 g

Marinated Green Beans

Preparation Time: 15 minutes

Serves 7

Serving Size: 1/2 cup

The tangy sauce perfectly perks up these green beans. I like my beans a little crisp. If you prefer them well done, choose the longer cooking period.

3 1/2 cups (3/4 lb) fresh green beans, trimmed and snapped

2 Tbsp chopped chives or thinly sliced green onion tops

2 Tbsp fat-free, low-sodium or regular chicken broth or bouillon

1 Tbsp catsup

1 Tbsp balsamic vinegar

2 tsp olive oil

1 tsp Dijon-style mustard

1/4 tsp salt, or to taste (optional)

2–3 drops hot pepper sauce

1. In a large saucepan, cook the beans in boiling water for 10 to 15 minutes until tender-crisp. Drain well in a colander.
2. Meanwhile, in a large bowl, combine the chives, broth, catsup, vinegar, oil, mustard, salt (if desired), and hot pepper sauce. Stir to mix well. Add the cooked beans, and stir to coat the beans with marinade.
3. Cover and refrigerate for 2 to 3 hours. Stir before serving. Leftover beans will keep in the refrigerator for 4 to 5 days.

Exchanges

1 Vegetable

Calories 30

Total Fat 1 g

Saturated Fat 0 g

Calories from Fat 13

Cholesterol 0 mg

Sodium 47 mg

Carbohydrate 4 g

Dietary Fiber 1 g

Sugars 1 g

Protein 1 g

Stuffed Celery Sticks

Preparation Time: 8 minutes

Serves 27

Serving Size: 1 celery stick

If you love the crunch of celery combined with a rich and flavorful filling, try this recipe.

4 oz Neufchâtel cream cheese

1/4 cup low-fat vanilla yogurt

1/2 cup water-packed crushed pineapple, well drained

1/2 cup grated or shredded carrot

2 Tbsp thinly sliced green onion tops

27 5-inch-long celery sticks

1. In a small bowl, stir together the Neufchâtel cheese and yogurt until well combined. Stir in the pineapple, carrot, and onion until well combined.
2. Fill each celery stick with 2 tsp of the mixture. The mixture can be used immediately or covered and refrigerated for up to 24 hours before using. The filling will keep, covered, in the refrigerator for 3 to 4 days.

Exchanges

Free

Calories 18

Total Fat 1 g

Saturated Fat 1 g

Calories from Fat 9

Cholesterol 3 mg

Sodium 35 mg

Carbohydrate 2 g

Dietary Fiber 0 g

Sugars 1 g

Protein 1 g

Salad Days

There's nothing like salads for a summer snack. Not only are they tasty, crunchy, and full of flavor, they're good for you, too, because they're packed with vitamins, minerals, and fiber. You'll find a great selection to choose from here. Some are old favorites, like Potato Salad. Others are my own creations, like Pasta, Bean, and Salmon Salad and Turkey Bulgur Salad. Some are simply vegetable combinations. Other add the taste and texture of grains and pasta, like my Carrot-Raisin Salad, which features the flavor and fiber of brown rice. All are made with dressings that are low in fat and calories.

Preparation Time: 18 minutes

Serves 5

Serving Size: 3/4 cup

Exchanges

1 Vegetable

1/2 Polyunsaturated Fat

Calories 51

Total Fat 2 g

Saturated Fat 0 g

Calories from Fat 18

Cholesterol 2 mg

Sodium 51 mg

Carbohydrate 8 g

Dietary Fiber 2 g

Sugars 5 g

Protein 1 g

Cabbage and Carrot Slaw

This yummy slaw has a great flavor and a pleasing, crunchy texture. And it's a wonderful way to increase your consumption of healthy vegetables. If you like, a small amount of sugar substitute could be used for the sugar in the recipe.

2 Tbsp cider vinegar

2 Tbsp reduced-fat mayonnaise

2 tsp sugar

1/4 tsp dry mustard

1/4 tsp salt, or to taste (optional)

1/8 tsp black pepper

4 cups very thinly sliced cabbage

1 large carrot, grated or shredded

1/2 red bell pepper, seeded and diced

1. In a large bowl, combine the vinegar, mayonnaise, sugar, mustard, salt (if desired), and black pepper. Whisk until well combined.
2. Add the cabbage, carrot, and pepper. Stir to coat the vegetables with dressing. Serve immediately, or cover and refrigerate. Leftover slaw will keep in the refrigerator 3 to 4 days.

Bean, Corn, and Rice Salad

Preparation Time: 10 minutes

Serves 9

Serving Size: 1/2 cup

You'll love the south-of-the-border flavor of this easy, hearty salad. The recipe calls for mild salsa. If you'd like more heat, substitute medium salsa for part of the mild. Brown rice varies considerably in consistency when cooked. Brands that remain firm and separate after cooking work best in this recipe.

3/4 cup mild low-sodium or regular salsa

1 Tbsp olive oil

1/2 tsp dried oregano leaves

1/4 tsp salt, or to taste (optional)

1 15-oz can low-sodium or regular kidney beans, rinsed and well drained

1 cup frozen corn kernels, cooked according to package directions

1 cup cooked brown rice

2 large celery stalks, diced

1. In a medium bowl, combine the salsa, oil, oregano, and salt (if desired). Stir to mix well.
2. Stir in the kidney beans, corn, rice, and celery. Mix well.
3. Serve at once, or cover and refrigerate. Leftover salad will keep in the refrigerator 3 to 4 days.

Exchanges

1 Starch

1/2 Monounsaturated Fat

Calories 104

Total Fat 2 g

Saturated Fat 0 g

Calories from Fat 18

Cholesterol 0 mg

Sodium 64 mg

Carbohydrate 18 g

Dietary Fiber 4 g

Sugars 3 g

Protein 4 g

Preparation Time: 15 minutes

Serves 7

Serving Size: 1/2 cup

Broccoli-Rice Salad

Here's a tasty way to enjoy broccoli. The recipe works best when made with a mild-flavored brown rice that holds its shape well after cooking.

4 cups small broccoli florets
3 Tbsp reduced-fat mayonnaise
1/4 cup low-fat buttermilk
2 tsp cider vinegar
1 tsp sugar
1/8 tsp ground celery seed
1/8 tsp white pepper
1/8 tsp salt, or to taste (optional)
1 cup cooked brown rice
2 Tbsp chopped red onion

1. To bring out the bright green color of the broccoli, place it in a medium saucepan with 1/4 cup water. Bring to a boil, and boil 1 minute. Remove from heat, and cool in a colander under cold running water. Drain.
2. Place the mayonnaise in a large serving bowl. Slowly add the buttermilk, whisking until smooth. Whisk in the vinegar, sugar, celery seed, pepper, and salt (if desired). Stir in the rice, reserved broccoli, and onion.
3. Serve at room temperature, or cover and refrigerate several hours. Leftover salad will keep in the refrigerator 2 to 3 days. Stir before serving.

Exchanges

1/2 Starch
1 Vegetable
1/2 Polyunsaturated Fat

Calories 71
Total Fat 2 g
Saturated Fat 0 g
Calories from Fat 22
Cholesterol 3 mg
Sodium 60 mg
Carbohydrate 11 g
Dietary Fiber 2 g
Sugars 3 g
Protein 2 g

Carrot-Raisin Salad

If you like the crunch and tang of traditional carrot-raisin salad, you'll love this version. The recipe calls for a teaspoon of optional honey, which enhances the sweetness of the carrots. But you could leave it out if you like.

2 Tbsp reduced-fat mayonnaise

1/4 cup low-fat buttermilk

1/2 Tbsp cider vinegar

1 tsp mild or strong honey (optional)

1 cup cooked brown rice

3 medium carrots, grated or shredded (1 cup)

1/3 cup dark raisins

1. Place the mayonnaise in a medium bowl. Slowly add the buttermilk, whisking until well combined. Whisk in the vinegar and honey (if desired).
2. Add the rice, carrots, and raisins, and stir to mix well.
3. Serve at once, or cover and refrigerate for several hours before serving. Leftover salad will keep in the refrigerator for 3 to 4 days.

Preparation Time: 12 minutes

Serves 4

Serving Size: 1/2 cup

Exchanges

1 Starch

1 Fruit

Calories 143

Total Fat 3 g

Saturated Fat 1 g

Calories from Fat 27

Cholesterol 4 mg

Sodium 76 mg

Carbohydrate 28 g

Dietary Fiber 2 g

Sugars 13 g

Protein 3 g

Preparation Time: 12 minutes

Serves 10

Serving Size: 1/2 cup

Exchanges

1 Starch

1/2 Monounsaturated Fat

Calories 100

Total Fat 2 g

Saturated Fat 0 g

Calories from Fat 17

Cholesterol 0 mg

Sodium 16 mg

Carbohydrate 17 g

Dietary Fiber 3 g

Sugars 2 g

Protein 4 g

Cajun Rice and Bean Salad

Here's a spicy New Orleans-style rice and bean salad. For best results, use brown rice that retains its shape after cooking.

1 cup low-sodium or regular stewed tomatoes

1 Tbsp olive oil

1/2 Tbsp cider vinegar

1/2 tsp dried marjoram leaves

1/2 tsp dried thyme leaves

1/4 tsp salt, or to taste (optional)

2–3 drops hot pepper sauce

2 cups cooked brown rice

1 15-oz can low-sodium or regular kidney beans, rinsed and well drained

1/4 cup thinly sliced green onion, including tops

1 large celery stalk, diced

1. In a medium bowl, combine the tomatoes, oil, vinegar, marjoram, thyme, salt (if desired), and hot pepper sauce. Stir to mix well.
2. Stir in the rice, beans, onion, and celery.
3. Serve the salad at room temperature, or cover and refrigerate before serving. Leftover salad will keep in the refrigerator 2 to 3 days.

Spanish Rice Salad

If you enjoy Spanish rice, try this salad variation.

2 cups cooked brown rice (about 1/2 cup uncooked)

1 Tbsp olive oil

1/2 Tbsp lemon juice

1 medium tomato, diced

1/2 sweet red pepper, seeded and diced

1/4 cup thinly sliced green onion, including tops

1/4 cup chopped fresh parsley

1 garlic clove, minced

1/4 tsp salt, or to taste (optional)

1. In a medium bowl, stir together the rice, olive oil, and lemon juice.
2. Stir in the tomato, pepper, onion, parsley, garlic, and salt (if desired). Mix well. Serve at room temperature, or cover and refrigerate several hours.
3. Leftover salad will keep in the refrigerator, covered, 3 to 4 days.

Preparation Time: 10 minutes

Serves 6

Serving Size: 1/2 cup

Exchanges

1 Starch

1/2 Monounsaturated Fat

Calories 105

Total Fat 3 g

Saturated Fat 1 g

Calories from Fat 27

Cholesterol 0 mg

Sodium 8 mg

Carbohydrate 18 g

Dietary Fiber 2 g

Sugars 2 g

Protein 2 g

Preparation Time: 12 minutes

Serves 4

Serving Size: 1/2 cup

Exchanges

1 1/2 Starch

1/2 Fat

Calories 135

Total Fat 6 g

Saturated Fat 1 g

Calories from Fat 51

Cholesterol 0 mg

Sodium 253 mg

Carbohydrate 21 g

Dietary Fiber 1 g

Sugars 2 g

Protein 4 g

Asian Noodles

The Chinese noodles called for in this recipe are the curly variety, similar to ramen noodles. They're available in specialty food markets and many grocery stores.

1/3 10-oz package Chinese noodles

1/4 cup fat-free, low-sodium or regular chicken broth

1 Tbsp smooth peanut butter

2 tsp light soy sauce

2 tsp Asian sesame oil

1 1/2 tsp rice or white vinegar

1/2 tsp ginger

3–4 drops hot pepper sauce

1/2 cup peeled and chopped broccoli stems

2 Tbsp chopped chives or sliced green onions

1. Cook the noodles according to the package directions. Rinse under cold water and drain in a colander. When the noodles are well drained, transfer to a medium bowl. Cut or tear long strands into smaller pieces.
2. In a small deep microwave-safe bowl, combine the broth, peanut butter, soy sauce, oil, vinegar, ginger, and hot pepper sauce. Microwave 20 to 30 seconds to warm the mixture so that the peanut butter will easily combine with other ingredients. With a small wire whisk, whisk until well combined. Stir in the broccoli and chives.
3. Stir the dressing mixture into the noodles. Serve warm, or cover and refrigerate. Leftover noodle salad will keep in the refrigerator for 3 to 4 days.

Pasta, Bean, and Salmon Salad

Quick and easy, this delicious salad can be made from ingredients that are probably in your pantry, and you can make the dressing and finish the rest of the preparations while the pasta is cooking.

Preparation Time: 11 minutes

Serves 8

Serving Size: 1/2 cup

3 Tbsp catsup

2 Tbsp cider vinegar

1 Tbsp olive oil

1 garlic clove, minced

1 tsp Italian seasoning

1/8 tsp salt, or to taste (optional)

1 cup uncooked penne or similarly shaped pasta

1 14 1/2-oz can low-sodium cut green beans, well drained

2 Tbsp chopped red onion or other sweet onion

1 6-oz can boneless, skinless pink salmon, well drained

1. In a large serving bowl, combine the catsup and vinegar. Stir to mix well. Stir in the oil, garlic, Italian seasoning, and salt (if desired). Set aside.
2. Cook the pasta according to package directions. Transfer to a colander and rinse under cold running water. Drain.
3. Meanwhile, add the green beans and onion to the bowl with the dressing. Stir to mix well. Stir in the pasta and salmon.
4. Serve immediately, or cover and refrigerate 1 hour or up to 36 hours before serving. Stir before serving. Leftover salad will keep in the refrigerator 3 to 4 days.

Exchanges

1/2 Starch

1 Lean Meat

Calories 100

Total Fat 3 g

Saturated Fat 0 g

Calories from Fat 28

Cholesterol 12 mg

Sodium 190 mg

Carbohydrate 12 g

Dietary Fiber 1 g

Sugars 2 g

Protein 6 g

Preparation Time: 16 minutes

Serves 10

Serving Size: 1/2 cup

Exchanges

1 Starch

Calories 81

Total Fat 3 g

Saturated Fat 1 g

Calories from Fat 25

Cholesterol 0 mg

Sodium 31 mg

Carbohydrate 13 g

Dietary Fiber 2 g

Sugars 2 g

Protein 2 g

Marinated Potato Salad

Potatoes that are just a little bit crisp work best in this zesty salad, since they hold together well when stirred into the dressing.

5 medium (about 1 1/2 lb) red-skinned potatoes, cut into 1/2-inch cubes

3 Tbsp fat-free, low-sodium or regular chicken broth

2 Tbsp olive oil

1 1/2 Tbsp plus 1 tsp balsamic vinegar

1 large celery stalk, thinly sliced

3 Tbsp chopped red onion or other sweet onion

1 1/2 tsp Dijon-style mustard

3/4 tsp basil

3/4 tsp dried thyme leaves

1/4 tsp salt, or to taste (optional)

2–3 drops hot pepper sauce

1. Combine the potatoes and enough water to cover in a large saucepan. Cover the pot and bring to a boil over high heat. Reduce the heat and simmer 6 to 11 minutes, until the potatoes are tender but not soft when pierced with a fork. Cool under cold running water. Drain well in a colander.
2. While the potatoes are cooking, in a large bowl or serving dish, combine the broth, oil, and vinegar. Stir to mix. Add the celery, onion, mustard, basil, thyme, salt (if desired), and hot pepper sauce. Stir to mix well.

3. To assemble the salad, add the potatoes, carefully stirring with a large spoon to coat them with the dressing mixture. Be careful not to break up the potatoes. Cover and refrigerate several hours, stirring occasionally, to allow flavors to blend. Leftover salad will keep for 3 to 4 days in the refrigerator.

Preparation Time:
15 minutes

Serves 12

Serving Size:
1/2 cup

Exchanges

1 Starch

Calories 68

Total Fat 2 g

Saturated Fat 0 g

Calories from Fat 15

Cholesterol 2 mg

Sodium 45 mg

Carbohydrate 12 g

Dietary Fiber 1 g

Sugars 2 g

Protein 2 g

Potato Salad

This potato salad has a tasty ranch-style dressing that combines reduced-fat mayonnaise and low-fat buttermilk. A number of steps will help you prepare this snack quickly. Cut up the potatoes before cooking them, and have the boiling water ready. Mix the dressing while the potatoes are cooking, and cool them quickly under cold running water.

5 cups (about 1 1/2 lb) red-skinned potatoes, cut into 3/4-inch cubes

1/4 cup reduced-fat mayonnaise

1/2 cup low-fat buttermilk

3/4 tsp basil

3/4 tsp dried thyme leaves

3/4 tsp dried marjoram leaves

1/8 tsp celery seed

1/4 tsp salt, or to taste (optional)

2–3 drops hot pepper sauce

1 small cucumber, peeled, seeded, and cubed

2 Tbsp chopped chives or green onions

1. In a small pot or very large saucepan, combine the potatoes with 1 quart of boiling water. Cover and bring to a boil again. Reduce the heat, and boil 9 to 14 minutes. Do not overcook. Cool in a colander under cold running water. Drain well.
2. Meanwhile, place the mayonnaise in a large serving bowl. Slowly add the buttermilk, whisking until smooth. Stir in the basil, thyme,

marjoram, celery seed, salt (if desired), and hot pepper sauce. Stir in the cucumber and chives. Gently stir in the cooled and drained potatoes.

3. Serve warm, or cover and refrigerate 1 or 2 hours, or cool in the freezer for 15 to 20 minutes. Cover and refrigerate. Leftover salad will keep in the refrigerator for 3 to 4 days.

Preparation Time: 18 minutes

Serves 16

Serving Size: 1/2 cup

Pasta-Vegetable Salad

If summer tomatoes are unavailable, substitute 5 or 6 Italian plum tomatoes. If you like, a small amount of sugar substitute could be used in place of the sugar in the recipe.

2 Tbsp cider vinegar

2 Tbsp tomato sauce

2 tsp sugar

2 Tbsp olive oil

1 garlic clove, minced

1/4 tsp dried marjoram leaves

1/4 tsp basil

1/4 tsp salt, or to taste (optional)

1 cup uncooked penne or similarly shaped pasta

1 large tomato, cubed

1 small zucchini, cubed

1 medium red or yellow pepper, seeded and chopped

1 cup broccoli or cauliflower florets

1. In a serving bowl, combine the vinegar and tomato sauce. Stir to mix well. Stir in the sugar, oil, garlic, marjoram, basil, and salt (if desired). Set aside.
2. Cook the pasta according to package directions. Transfer to a colander and rinse under cold running water. Drain.
3. Meanwhile, add the tomatoes, zucchini, pepper, and broccoli to the bowl with the dressing. Stir to mix well. Stir in pasta. Serve immediately, or cover and refrigerate 1 hour or up to 36 hours before serving. Stir before serving.

Exchanges

1/2 Starch

Calories 44

Total Fat 2 g

Saturated Fat 0 g

Calories from Fat 17

Cholesterol 0 mg

Sodium 14 mg

Carbohydrate 6 g

Dietary Fiber 1 g

Sugars 2 g

Protein 1 g

Three-Bean Snack

Try this quick and easy variation of the popular three-bean salad.

1/4 cup chili sauce

3 Tbsp fat-free, low-sodium or regular chicken broth

1 1/2 Tbsp red wine vinegar

1 Tbsp olive oil

2 tsp Italian seasoning

2–3 drops hot pepper sauce

1/4 tsp salt, or to taste (optional)

1 16-oz can low-sodium or regular kidney beans, rinsed and well drained

1 14 1/2-oz can wax beans, rinsed and well drained

1 14 1/2-oz can low-sodium or regular cut green beans, rinsed and well drained

2 Tbsp chopped red onion or other sweet onion

1. In a large bowl, combine the chili sauce, broth, vinegar, oil, Italian seasoning, hot pepper sauce, and salt (if desired). Stir to mix well.
2. Add the beans and onion, and stir gently to coat with the dressing.
3. Serve at once or cover and refrigerate. Leftover salad will keep in the refrigerator 3 to 4 days.

Preparation Time: 10 minutes

Serves 8

Serving Size: 1/2 cup

Exchanges

1/2 Starch

1 Vegetable

1/2 Monounsaturated Fat

Calories 80

Total Fat 2 g

Saturated Fat 0 g

Calories from Fat 17

Cholesterol 0 mg

Sodium 260 mg

Carbohydrate 12 g

Dietary Fiber 4 g

Sugars 3 g

Protein 4 g

Preparation Time: 11 minutes

Serves 9

Serving Size: 1/2 cup

Exchanges

1/2 Starch

1/2 Monounsaturated Fat

Calories 63

Total Fat 3 g

Saturated Fat 1 g

Calories from Fat 30

Cholesterol 2 mg

Sodium 102 mg

Carbohydrate 7 g

Dietary Fiber 1 g

Sugars 2 g

Protein 2 g

Italian Bread Salad

The Italians invented this chunky salad as a way to use up stale bread. I prefer lightly toasted whole-wheat bread cut into cubes.

3 Tbsp fat-free, low-sodium or regular chicken broth

2 Tbsp grated Parmesan cheese

1 1/2 Tbsp olive oil

1 Tbsp red wine vinegar

1/8 tsp salt (optional)

1/8 tsp black pepper

1 1/2 cups (about 15–25) cherry tomatoes, sliced in half before measuring

1 medium cucumber, peeled, seeded, and cubed

2 Tbsp thinly sliced chives or green onion tops

2 Tbsp chopped fresh basil leaves or 1/4 tsp dried basil leaves

2 cups 1/2-inch bread cubes

1. In a 2-cup measure or similar deep bowl, combine the broth, cheese, oil, vinegar, salt (if desired), and pepper. Stir briskly with a fork to mix well. Set aside.
2. In a medium salad bowl, mix together the tomato, cucumber, chives, and fresh basil. (If using dried basil, mix it into the salad dressing.)
3. Pour the dressing over the vegetables and toss to mix. Add the bread cubes and thoroughly toss to coat them with dressing. Serve at once. This salad will keep for a day in the refrigerator, although the bread tends to absorb the dressing.

Tabouli

This traditional Middle Eastern salad is filling and flavorful.

Preparation Time: 30 minutes

Serves 6

Serving Size: 1/2 cup

1 cup dry bulgur wheat

1 1/2 cups boiling water

2 Tbsp lemon juice

2 Tbsp olive oil

2 garlic cloves, minced

1 tsp salt, or to taste (optional)

2–3 drops hot pepper sauce (optional)

1/4 cup sliced green onion tops

2 Tbsp fresh mint leaves or 1/2 tsp dried mint

1/2 cup coarsely chopped fresh parsley

1 large tomato, diced

1 small cucumber, peeled, seeded, and diced

1. In a large bowl, combine the bulgur and boiling water. Cover and let stand 15 to 20 minutes, until the bulgur has softened and most of the water has been absorbed. Drain in a sieve. Return the bulgur to the bowl.
2. Add the lemon juice, oil, garlic, salt (if desired), and hot pepper sauce (if desired). Stir to mix well. Stir in the onions, mint, parsley, tomato, and cucumber. Stir the vegetable mixture into the bulgur.
3. Serve at once, or cover and refrigerate several hours. Stir before serving. Leftover tabouli will keep in the refrigerator for 2 to 3 days.

Exchanges

1 Starch

1 Vegetable

1/2 Monounsaturated Fat

Calories 135

Total Fat 5 g

Saturated Fat 1 g

Calories from Fat 45

Cholesterol 0 mg

Sodium 12 mg

Carbohydrate 21 g

Dietary Fiber 5 g

Sugars 2 g

Protein 4 g

Preparation Time: 30 minutes

Serves 4

Serving Size: 1/2 cup

Turkey Bulgur Salad

1/2 cup bulgur wheat

1 cup boiling water

2 Tbsp fat-free, low-sodium or regular chicken broth

1 Tbsp olive oil

1/2 Tbsp lemon juice

1/2 tsp dried thyme leaves

1/2 tsp dry mustard

3/4 cup (3 oz) cooked turkey breast, cut into small pieces

1 celery stalk, chopped

1/4 cup red bell pepper, seeded and chopped

2 Tbsp chopped fresh parsley

2 Tbsp red onion, minced

1/4 tsp salt, or to taste (optional)

Dash black pepper

1. In a medium bowl, combine the bulgur and boiling water. Cover and let stand 15 to 20 minutes, until the bulgur has softened and most of the water has been absorbed. Drain in a sieve. Return the bulgur to the bowl.
2. While the bulgur is softening, in a medium bowl, combine the broth, oil, lemon juice, thyme, and dry mustard. Stir to mix well.
3. Stir in the turkey, celery, red pepper, parsley, onion, salt (if desired), and pepper.
4. Stir the turkey mixture into the softened bulgur. Serve at once, or cover and refrigerate several hours. Stir before serving. Leftover salad will keep in the refrigerator 2 to 3 days.

Exchanges

1 Starch

1 Lean Meat

Calories 127

Total Fat 4 g

Saturated Fat 1 g

Calories from Fat 34

Cholesterol 17 mg

Sodium 48 mg

Carbohydrate 15 g

Dietary Fiber 4 g

Sugars 1 g

Protein 9 g

Turkey Salad with Apples and Almonds

You'll love this variation of a classic chicken salad! This recipe calls for toasting the almonds, which adds wonderful flavor to the salad.

Preparation Time: 16 minutes

Serves 4

Serving Size: 1/2 cup

2 Tbsp sliced almonds

3 Tbsp fat-free sour cream

1 Tbsp reduced-fat mayonnaise

Dash ground celery seed

Dash ground cardamom

1/8 tsp salt or to taste (optional)

1 cup (5 oz) roasted turkey or chicken breast cubes

1 cup cubed tart or sweet apple, peeled or unpeeled

1 small celery stalk, diced

1. Spray a medium nonstick skillet with nonstick spray. Add the almonds. Over medium heat, cook the almonds, stirring, until they brown and smell toasted, about 4 or 5 minutes. If the almonds begin to burn, lower the heat slightly. Immediately remove to a small plate and set aside.
2. In a medium bowl, stir together the sour cream, mayonnaise, celery seed, cardamom, and salt (if desired).
3. Stir in the turkey, apple, celery, and reserved almonds. Serve at once, or cover and refrigerate several hours or up to 24 hours. Leftover salad will keep in the refrigerator for 2 to 3 days.

Exchanges

1/2 Carbohydrate

1 Lean Meat

Calories 111

Total Fat 3 g

Saturated Fat 0 g

Calories from Fat 30

Cholesterol 30 mg

Sodium 78 mg

Carbohydrate 8 g

Dietary Fiber 2 g

Sugars 6 g

Protein 12 g

Preparation Time: 15 minutes

Serves 5

Serving Size: 1/2 cup

Curried Turkey Salad

Curry and pineapple make a wonderful foil for the turkey breast meat in this salad. You can buy a turkey breast and roast it at home, reserving the remaining meat for another purpose. Or you can buy thick-cut roasted turkey breast from a deli or a package of roasted turkey breast meat.

1/2 cup juice-packed crushed pineapple, well drained
1/4 cup fat-free sour cream
2 Tbsp reduced-fat mayonnaise
1 tsp mild curry powder
1/4 tsp salt, or to taste (optional)
1 cup (5 oz) cubed turkey breast meat
1 8-oz can sliced water chestnuts, well drained
1 small celery stalk, chopped
2 Tbsp chopped chives or sliced green onion tops

1. In a medium bowl, stir together the pineapple, sour cream, mayonnaise, curry powder, and salt (if desired).
2. Stir in the turkey, water chestnuts, celery, and chives. Serve at once, or cover and refrigerate several hours or up to 24 hours. Leftover salad will keep in the refrigerator for 2 to 3 days.

Exchanges

1/2 Fruit

1 Vegetable

1 Very Lean Meat

Calories 97

Total Fat 2 g

Saturated Fat 0 g

Calories from Fat 19

Cholesterol 25 mg

Sodium 89 mg

Carbohydrate 10 g

Dietary Fiber 1 g

Sugars 6 g

Protein 10 g

Just For Kids

The recipes in this chapter are fun to make and fun to munch! Many, like my Pear Mice, Celery Man, and Alphabet Letters, are designed to get little kids interested in eating the fruits and vegetables that are so good for them. Others are fanciful interpretations of the sandwich theme. And there are two sweet and crunchy popcorn snacks that go easy on the syrup.

While these recipes are designed especially for kids, there are a lot of others elsewhere in this book, like my Egg 'N Muffin, Turkey Salad Sandwich, or Pizza Puffs, that make great after-school snacks. Other kid pleasers include Cheese Popcorn, Cranberry Orange Muffins, and Carrot-Raisin Salad.

On the other hand, my adult friends have enjoyed many of the recipes in this chapter, too. So don't think you have to be a kid to try snacks like French Toast Bites, Caramel Apples, Cinnamon Triangles, or a Banana Pop.

Preparation Time:
10 minutes

Serves 1

Celery Man

Here's a whimsical vegetable man who's fun to eat.

1 large celery stalk with some leaves, if possible
2 raisins
1 dried cranberry
1 Tbsp cottage cheese spread (see recipe, p. 5), plain low-fat cottage cheese, flavored fat-free yogurt, or canned shredded beets

1. To make the man, lay a large celery stalk on a flat surface with the leafy part facing away from you and the concave side up. The leaves and stem pieces above the joint will be the hair. The next inch of stalk will be the head.
2. To make the head stand out from the body, create a neck by carving two shallow half-moon shapes into the sides of the stalk. For the arms, carefully cut two long slivers at the sides of the stalk below the neck. Gently pull the arms to a 45-degree angle from the body, being careful not to detach them.
3. For the legs, make a 3- or 4-inch cut from the bottom of the stalk toward the top. Gently open the legs slightly, being careful not to detach them.
4. To make the face, use two raisins for eyes and a dried cranberry for a mouth. Dress the body of the man by spooning on 1 Tbsp of desired spread or topping.

Exchanges

1 Vegetable

Calories 29
Total Fat 0 g
Saturated Fat 0 g
Calories from Fat 3
Cholesterol 1 mg
Sodium 109 mg
Carbohydrate 4 g
Dietary Fiber 1 g
Sugars 3 g
Protein 2 g

Pear Mice

Preparation Time: 6 minutes

Serves 1

Here's a fun way to enjoy pear salad—turn pear halves into cute little mice. The recipe gives one garnishing suggestion. But you could also use cut strawberries for ears, a piece of cooked pasta for a tail, and a raisin for a nose.

2 juice-packed canned pear halves

4 currants (or 2 dark raisins cut in half and rounded)

1 dried cranberry, cut in half

2 grapes, cut in half lengthwise (or two golden raisins, flattened)

2 3-inch slivers of sweet pepper or celery

1. Lay the pear halves, cut side down, on a plate. You can position both pieces with the narrow end facing either toward you or away from you, or one of each. The narrow end of the pear will be the face and the big end will be the body.
2. To turn a pear half into a mouse, lay half a dried cranberry at the tip of the narrow end for a nose. Press two currants into place above the nose for eyes. Make the ears of grape halves, set in place on either side of the head. If necessary, cut small slits in the pear flesh to hold the ears erect.
3. To make the tail, lay a sliver of sweet pepper or celery at the large end of the mouse. Repeat with the second pear half.

Exchanges

1 1/2 Fruit

Calories 77

Total Fat 0 g

Saturated Fat 0 g

Calories from Fat 2

Cholesterol 0 mg

Sodium 5 mg

Carbohydrate 20 g

Dietary Fiber 3 g

Sugars 15 g

Protein 1 g

Preparation Time: 10 minutes

Serves 1

Mr. and Mrs. Pear Head

Mr. and Mrs. Pear Head are a fun addition to afternoon snack time. You can use a variety of fruit and vegetable pieces to make the eyes, nose, mouth, and hair. Below are several suggestions, but you could also use a cut piece of strawberry for the mouth, red grapes for eyes, and currants or pieces of dried apricot for various features. For variety, try shredded lettuce or shoe-string beets for hair. Either the narrow end or the wide end of the pear can be the top of the head.

2 juice-packed canned pear halves

4 raisins

2 carrot half circles

1/4 cup grated carrot or crushed pineapple

1. Lay the pear halves, cut side down, on a plate.
2. Give the pear halves eyes and mouths. Use two raisins for eyes on each pair half, and press them into place. Place the carrot half circles into place for the mouths.
3. For hair, arrange grated carrot or crushed pineapple on the plate at the top of the head. Or give Mrs. Pear Head all the hair and leave her husband bald.

Exchanges

1 Fruit

1 Vegetable

Calories 85

Total Fat 0 g

Saturated Fat 0 g

Calories from Fat 2

Cholesterol 0 mg

Sodium 19 mg

Carbohydrate 22 g

Dietary Fiber 4 g

Sugars 16 g

Protein 1 g

Dugout Canoes

Preparation Time: 6 minutes

Serves 2

Serving Size: 1 canoe

It's fun to remove the seeds from a cucumber and fill the cavity with vegetable stick logs. Or fill with Tuna Salad (p. 12), Salmon Salad (p. 11), Turkey Salad (p. 39), or Cottage Cheese with Dill and Onion (p. 5; the nutritional analysis was calculated using this filling).

1 medium cucumber

1 carrot, cut into sticks

1 celery stalk, cut into 2-inch sections

1 Tbsp filling of choice (optional, see suggestions above)

1. With a vegetable peeler, remove the skin from the cucumber. Lay the cucumber on a flat surface, and cut in half lengthwise.
2. With a teaspoon, carefully scrape the seeds from the cucumber and discard them.
3. Fill with carrot and celery sticks or filling of choice.

Exchanges

1 Vegetable

Calories 30

Total Fat 0 g

Saturated Fat 0 g

Calories from Fat 4

Cholesterol 1 mg

Sodium 88 mg

Carbohydrate 3 g

Dietary Fiber 2 g

Sugars 4 g

Protein 2 g

Preparation Time:
8 minutes

Serves 1

Mad Teacup

This fruit cup was inspired by the mad spinning teacup rides we've all enjoyed at many amusement parks. If you want to recreate the whirling motion by spinning your plate, do it carefully!

1/2 medium apple, cored

1/2 tsp lemon juice

1 juice-packed pineapple ring

1/4 cup berries or diced fruit

Mint sprig (optional)

1. With a teaspoon or small knife, carefully dig out some of the apple flesh so that the half apple forms a cup. Rub the lemon juice over the apple surface.
2. Place the pineapple ring on a small plate. Set the apple in the center of the ring. Fill the apple center with berries or diced fruit. Garnish with a sprig of mint, if you like.

Exchanges

1 Fruit

Calories 73

Total Fat 0 g

Saturated Fat 0 g

Calories from Fat 4

Cholesterol 0 mg

Sodium 1 mg

Carbohydrate 19 g

Dietary Fiber 3 g

Sugars 15 g

Protein 0 g

Egg Sailboats

Preparation Time: 3 minutes

Serves 1

These cute little egg sailboats skim across the plate. (In fact, it would be fun to serve them on a blue paper plate.) The yolks are removed and replaced with a healthier filling, such as Tuna Salad (p. 12; the nutritional analysis was calculated using this filling), Turkey Salad (p. 39), or the Deviled Egg Mixture (p. 43). Use a triangle cut from a cabbage leaf, a sweet pepper, or a piece of spinach for the sail. Or, for an interesting variation, omit the sail and fill the cavity with Guacamole Dip (p. 9) or mashed green peas, and call them "green eggs." You could even serve them with a thin slice of low-fat deli ham!

1 hard-cooked large egg

1 Tbsp filling of choice (see suggestions above)

1 2-inch-high triangle cut from a cabbage or spinach leaf or a piece of sweet pepper

1. Cut the egg in half, and scoop out and discard the yolk. Fill the cavity with filling of choice.
2. Stick a vegetable triangle into the top of the filling to serve as a sail for the egg boat.

Exchanges

1 Very Lean Meat

Calories 41

Total Fat 1 g

Saturated Fat 0 g

Calories from Fat 8

Cholesterol 5 mg

Sodium 114 mg

Carbohydrate 1 g

Dietary Fiber 0 g

Sugars 1 g

Protein 7 g

Preparation Time: 15 minutes

Serves 2

Serving Size: 1 cup

Exchanges

1 Vegetable

1/2 Fat

Calories 42

Total Fat 2 g

Saturated Fat 0 g

Calories from Fat 16

Cholesterol 0 mg

Sodium 116 mg

Carbohydrate 9 g

Dietary Fiber 3 g

Sugars 5 g

Protein 1 g

Alphabet Letters

How many letters of the alphabet can you make from vegetable pieces? How many words? It's fun to find out! Straight pieces cut from vegetables like celery, carrot, zucchini, and green beans can form many letters, such as A, T, E, F, and H. Carrot, zucchini, and cucumber circles and half circles make the curves of letters like B, C, D, and O. Use a colorful mixture of vegetables to create letters and words.

30 straight vegetable pieces, about 2 inches long and 1/4 inch wide, cut from celery, carrot, cucumber, zucchini, red pepper, green pepper, and green beans

20 vegetable circles and half circles cut from carrot, cucumber, zucchini, and yellow squash

2 Tbsp reduced-fat salad dressing

1. Serve the vegetable pieces on two separate plates—one for straight pieces and one for rounds. Select from the pieces to make letters of the alphabet and words.
2. Decorate the finished letters and words with salad dressing, and eat!

Vegetable Centipede

Preparation Time: 12 minutes

Serves 1

Make raw vegetables into a creepy, crawly critter with this fun-to-eat centipede. You can also use a broccoli or cauliflower floret or a large radish for the critter's head and zucchini or yellow squash rounds for the body. Try cutting orange eyes from a piece of carrot or red eyes from a sweet red pepper. It works best to pick contrasting colors for the body and the legs.

7 carrot, cucumber, or cooked beet circles

12 celery or carrot sticks, about 2 inches long and 1/3 inch wide

2 fresh or frozen green peas

2 thin celery pieces

1 green onion, root trimmed so that about an inch of green top is left attached to the white part

1 Tbsp reduced-fat salad dressing

1. On a large plate, lay the circle pieces in a line, one behind the other to form the body of the centipede, curving the line slightly, if desired. Use the largest circle for the head at the top of the line. Arrange the celery or carrot sticks so that they stick out at right angles on either side of the body segments to form legs. (There will be no legs on the head segment.)
2. Arrange two peas on the head segment for eyes. Position two thin celery pieces for antennae. Make vertical cuts in the green top of the onion to create a brush-like effect. Fan out the brush to form a tail, and lay it below the last segment. Let the snacker decorate the centipede with salad dressing.

Exchanges

1 Vegetable

1/2 Fat

Calories 56

Total Fat 3 g

Saturated Fat 1 g

Calories from Fat 28

Cholesterol 4 mg

Sodium 134 mg

Carbohydrate 6 g

Dietary Fiber 2 g

Sugars 3 g

Protein 1 g

Preparation Time: 6 minutes

Serves 10

Serving Size: 1 cup

Exchanges

1/2 Carbohydrate

Calories 53

Total Fat 1 g

Saturated Fat 0 g

Calories from Fat 7

Cholesterol 1 mg

Sodium 59 mg

Carbohydrate 11 g

Dietary Fiber 1 g

Sugars 6 g

Protein 1 g

Easy Caramel Popcorn

The directions call for finishing this easy popcorn snack by baking it to harden the syrup. If you don't mind sticky popcorn, you can skip the baking step. In any case, be sure to cool the popcorn before serving, as hot syrup can burn your mouth.

10 cups popped low-fat microwave popcorn

6 caramel candies, cut into small pieces

2 Tbsp dark or light corn syrup

1/2 Tbsp water

1. Preheat the oven to 350 degrees. Spray a large jelly roll pan or rimmed cookie sheet with nonstick spray coating, and set aside. Place the popcorn in a large ceramic or glass bowl, and set aside.
2. In a 1-cup measure or similar microwave-safe bowl, combine the caramels, syrup, and water. Cover with wax paper and microwave on high power for 40 seconds. Stir. Microwave for an additional 30 seconds until the caramels are completely melted.
3. Being very careful to keep fingers away from the hot syrup, slowly pour the caramel mixture over the popcorn, stirring with a large wooden spoon to coat evenly. Spread the popcorn evenly on the prepared baking pan. Bake the popcorn for 4 to 6 minutes until the syrup hardens slightly.
4. Cool before serving, or store tightly covered at room temperature. Leftover popcorn will keep for 4 to 5 days.

Popcorn Crunch

Preparation Time: 20 minutes

Serves 10

Serving Size: 1 cup

Coating popcorn with syrup is a great way to satisfy a sweet tooth, since it makes a little syrup go a long way. Check nutritional labels on microwave popcorn, as some brands have more fat than others.

10 cups popped low-fat microwave popcorn

1/3 cup sugar

3 Tbsp molasses

1 Tbsp water

1 tsp vanilla extract

1. Spray a very large (at least 10 1/2- by 13 1/2-inch) baking pan with nonstick spray. Set aside. Preheat the oven to 375 degrees. Remove and discard unpopped kernels from popcorn. Set popcorn aside.
2. In a small saucepan, combine the sugar, molasses, and water, and stir to mix well. Cook over medium-high heat, stirring with a wooden spoon, until the mixture comes to a full boil. Boil, stirring constantly, 1 minute.
3. Remove from heat. With a wooden spoon, stir in vanilla until completely combined. Very slowly drizzle the syrup over the popcorn, stirring well to coat evenly and keeping fingers away from hot syrup.
4. Spread the popcorn evenly in the pan. Bake on center oven rack for 5 to 6 minutes until the popcorn begins to crisp slightly. Remove from the oven and stir. Cool. Syrup will harden, and popcorn will crisp further as it cools. When cool, store in a sealed plastic bag or airtight container for 2 to 3 days.

Exchanges

1 Carbohydrate

Calories 72

Total Fat 1 g

Saturated Fat 0 g

Calories from Fat 7

Cholesterol 0 mg

Sodium 3 mg

Carbohydrate 17 g

Dietary Fiber 1 g

Sugars 10 g

Protein 1 g

Preparation Time: 6 minutes

Serves 2

Serving Size: 1/2 apple

Caramel Apples

Caramel and apple make a great combination! This easy variation calls for cored apple cut into pieces and stirred into the syrup. An added advantage is that you can make this recipe with very little candy.

2 1/2 caramel candies, cut into small pieces

1/2 Tbsp dark or light corn syrup

1 large tart apple, cored and cut into bite-sized pieces

1. In a 1-cup measure or similar microwave-safe bowl, combine the caramels and corn syrup. Microwave on high power for 30 seconds. Stir and microwave for 15 additional seconds, or until the caramels are completely melted.
2. Stir well, and mix in the apple pieces, stirring to coat them with syrup. Cool slightly. Divide into two servings. Eat with a fork.

Exchanges

2 Carbohydrate

Calories 120

Total Fat 1 g

Saturated Fat 1 g

Calories from Fat 11

Cholesterol 1 mg

Sodium 35 mg

Carbohydrate 28 g

Dietary Fiber 3 g

Sugars 22 g

Protein 1 g

French Toast Bites

Preparation Time: 5 minutes

Serves 2

Serving Size: 1 piece

Serve these kid-sized French toast squares for breakfast or a snack. Top them with mashed banana, crushed pineapple, a little Pear or Apple Spread (pages 157 and 158), some low-fat vanilla yogurt, or some sugar-free pancake syrup.

2 slices whole-wheat or cracked wheat bread
1/4 cup liquid egg substitute
3 Tbsp low-fat (1%) milk
1/4 tsp vanilla extract
Pinch cinnamon or nutmeg
Pinch salt (optional)

1. Cut each bread slice into 4 squares or triangles. In a medium shallow bowl or flat casserole, stir together the egg substitute, milk, vanilla, cinnamon, and salt (if desired).
2. Add the bread. With a large flat spoon or narrow blade spatula, gently move the squares around slightly to help them absorb the liquid. When about half the liquid has been absorbed, turn them and repeat the process until most of the egg mixture is used up.
3. Transfer the squares to a large nonstick spray-coated nonstick skillet preheated over medium heat. Brown each slice for 3 to 4 minutes, turning each over once with a narrow blade spatula during cooking. Serve plain or with a desired topping.

Exchanges

1 Starch

Calories 96
Total Fat 1 g
Saturated Fat 0 g
Calories from Fat 13
Cholesterol 1 mg
Sodium 214 mg
Carbohydrate 15 g
Dietary Fiber 2 g
Sugars 2 g
Protein 7 g

Preparation Time: 15 minutes

Serves 2

Serving Size: 1/2 bagel

Holiday Wreaths

Here's a fun way to observe the holiday season—with wreaths made from a bagel. It's surprising how much these edible wreaths look like the real thing. The recipe calls for dried chopped cranberries. If you like, you can use part cranberries and part chopped dried apricot for a multicolored effect.

1 whole-wheat or plain bagel

2 Tbsp Neufchâtel low-fat cream cheese

3 Tbsp finely chopped fresh parsley leaves

1 tsp dried cranberries, chopped

1. Cut the bagel in half, and lay each half on a plate. Spread each bagel half with half the cream cheese.
2. Sprinkle the parsley evenly over the cream cheese and press into place. Attractively arrange chopped cranberries on the surface of the wreath.

Exchanges

1 1/2 Starch

1/2 Saturated Fat

Calories 139

Total Fat 4 g

Saturated Fat 2 g

Calories from Fat 33

Cholesterol 10 mg

Sodium 253 mg

Carbohydrate 21 g

Dietary Fiber 1 g

Sugars 3 g

Protein 5 g

Bread Puzzle

Here's the perfect snack for kids who like to play with their food—a bread slice puzzle! (Hint: To make it easy to spread refrigerated peanut butter, scoop it out of the jar with a plastic measuring spoon. Then lay the spoon in a microwave oven, and microwave on high power 5 to 10 seconds.)

Preparation Time: 7 minutes

Serves 1

1 slice whole-wheat bread, toasted

1/2 Tbsp peanut butter

1 Tbsp homemade Apple Spread (p. 158) or mashed banana or crushed juice-packed pineapple

1. Lay the toast slice on a cutting board. With a small, sharp knife, cut the bread into 2, 3, or 4 sections with tabs sticking from one section into the other, so that the pieces form a puzzle. Or cut a stair-step effect down the center of the bread slice. (It's easier to cut straight lines than curves.) Carefully separate the pieces to make sure they come apart.
2. Lay the puzzle pieces back in the original bread slice shape. Spread the sections with peanut butter and other desired topping. Mix up puzzle pieces and fit them back together before eating.

Exchanges

1 1/2 Starch

1/2 Monounsaturated Fat

Calories 137

Total Fat 5 g

Saturated Fat 1 g

Calories from Fat 48

Cholesterol 0 mg

Sodium 185 mg

Carbohydrate 20 g

Dietary Fiber 3 g

Sugars 7 g

Protein 5 g

Preparation Time: 15 minutes

Serves 2

Serving Size: 1 slice

At the Zoo

Make snack time fun with an edible zoo, using toasted bread and cookie cutters. Or try other shapes for various holidays: hearts for Valentine's Day; stars, trees, and bells for the winter holidays; and shamrocks for St. Patrick's Day.

2–3 slices whole-wheat bread, toasted

1 Tbsp peanut butter or Neufchâtel cheese

1 Tbsp homemade Pear or Apple Spread (pp. 157 and 158) or 2 Tbsp mashed banana or 2 Tbsp crushed juice-packed pineapple

Raisins, currants, or dried apricots (optional)

1. Press the cookie cutters firmly into the toasted bread to make an animal or other shape. Spread with one or two of the suggested toppings. For even more fun, use raisins or currants for eyes and noses and a sliver of dried apricot for a mouth.
2. If you're making shamrocks, you can spread clover shapes with Neufchâtel and cover with finely chopped parsley leaves. You can use the same technique for a holiday tree, and decorate it with raisins, dried cranberries, and chopped dried fruit. For hearts, mix a little red food coloring and a dash of cinnamon into Neufchâtel.

Exchanges

1 Starch

1/2 Monounsaturated Fat

Calories 107

Total Fat 5 g

Saturated Fat 1 g

Calories from Fat 45

Cholesterol 0 mg

Sodium 148 mg

Carbohydrate 13 g

Dietary Fiber 2 g

Sugars 3 g

Protein 4 g

Hawaiian Pizza

Here's a fun "pizza" made with fruit instead of tomato sauce and cheese.

1 whole-wheat or oat bran English muffin or 2 small whole-wheat pita bread rounds

1/4 cup fat-free vanilla yogurt

1/3 cup sliced fresh strawberries

3 Tbsp juice-packed crushed pineapple, well-drained

1. Toast the muffin halves. Spread with the yogurt.
2. Spoon the strawberries on the muffin halves. Sprinkle with the crushed pineapple.

Preparation Time: 5 minutes

Serves 2

Serving Size: 1 piece

Exchanges

1 Starch

1/2 Fruit

Calories 95

Total Fat 1 g

Saturated Fat 0 g

Calories from Fat 8

Cholesterol 1 mg

Sodium 128 mg

Carbohydrate 19 g

Dietary Fiber 2 g

Sugars 7 g

Protein 4 g

Preparation Time: 3 minutes

Serves 2

Serving Size: 1 piece

Aladdin's Pizza

Aladdin would have loved these easy fruit and yogurt pizzas, which can also be made on toasted whole-wheat English muffin halves.

2 small pita bread rounds

1/4 cup reduced-fat vanilla yogurt

2 Tbsp chopped dried fruit, such as apricots, raisins, apples, or pears

1. Spread the pita bread rounds with yogurt.
2. Sprinkle with fruit. Serve immediately.

Exchanges

1 Starch

1 Fruit

Calories 145

Total Fat 1 g

Saturated Fat 0 g

Calories from Fat 8

Cholesterol 3 mg

Sodium 179 mg

Carbohydrate 31 g

Dietary Fiber 2 g

Sugars 12 g

Protein 4 g

Cinnamon Triangles

Preparation Time: 6 minutes

Serves 6

Serving Size: 5 triangles

Fun and easy to fix, these crispy treats are made with purchased wonton wrappers.

2 tsp sugar

1/8 tsp cinnamon

15 wonton wrappers

1 1/2 tsp reduced-fat tubstyle margarine (4.5 g fat/T)

1. Preheat the oven to 400 degrees. Spray a small baking sheet with nonstick spray coating. Set aside.
2. In a custard cup, mix together the sugar and cinnamon. Cut 15 wonton wrappers in half to form triangles, and lay them on the baking sheet.
3. With your finger or the back of a spoon, brush the top of each wrapper with margarine, dividing it evenly. Sprinkle the cinnamon-sugar mixture over the top of each wrapper, dividing evenly.
4. Bake in the center of the oven for 3 to 4 minutes or until golden. Cool slightly before serving. Leftovers can be wrapped tightly and kept at room temperature for up to a week.

Exchanges

1/2 Starch

Calories 51

Total Fat 1 g

Saturated Fat 0 g

Calories from Fat 6

Cholesterol 3 mg

Sodium 93 mg

Carbohydrate 10 g

Dietary Fiber 1 g

Sugars 2 g

Protein 2 g

Preparation Time: 8 minutes

Serves 8

Serving Size: 1 turnover

Over-Easy Apple-Raisin Turnovers

1 1/2 tsp sugar

1/8 tsp cinnamon

1 medium apple, peeled or unpeeled, cored and cut into small cubes

1 Tbsp dark raisins

8 very fresh, reduced-calorie, whole-wheat bread slices

1. In a custard cup, or on a small sheet of wax paper, stir together the sugar and cinnamon. In a 2-cup measure or similar small microwave-safe bowl, combine the sugar-cinnamon mixture, apple, and raisins. Stir to mix well.
2. Cover with wax paper and microwave on high power for 1 minute. Stir. Re-cover and microwave on high power an additional 1 to 1 1/2 minutes or until the apples are softened. Meanwhile, trim the crusts from the bread slices and discard them. With a rolling pin, flatten the slices to 1/8 inch thick.
3. Place a generous tablespoon of apple mixture on one side of each bread slice, and spread it out slightly. To form turnovers, fold the bread over the filling to make a triangle shape. Seal the edges by pressing with fork tines.
4. Lightly toast the slices in the toaster oven. Or toast under the broiler, browning lightly on one side and then the other. Cool slightly before eating. You can make up a batch of filling, use some of it immediately, and save the rest in the refrigerator. Then make additional turnovers over the next 2 to 3 days.

Exchanges

1/2 Carbohydrate

Calories 47

Total Fat 0 g

Saturated Fat 0 g

Calories from Fat 2

Cholesterol 0 mg

Sodium 75 mg

Carbohydrate 11 g

Dietary Fiber 2 g

Sugars 5 g

Protein 2 g

Banana Pops

Preparation Time: 3 minutes

Serves 6

Serving Size: 1 pop

Frozen banana pops are a snap to make and taste a lot like ice cream. For extra pizzazz, drizzle them with chocolate syrup before serving. The recipe calls for using popsicle sticks. If they are unavailable, the end of each pop can be held in a folded piece of plastic wrap.

6 small ripe bananas
6 popsicle sticks
6 Tbsp chocolate syrup (optional)

1. For each pop, carefully insert a popsicle stick into the bottom of 1 banana, burying about half of the stick. Wrap each banana individually in plastic wrap, and freeze for at least 6 hours.
2. To serve, unwrap each banana, and eat like a popsicle. If desired, lay each banana on a plate, and drizzle with 1 Tbsp of chocolate syrup before serving. To combat dripping chocolate, hold the pop over the plate while eating it.
3. Frozen banana pops will keep in the freezer, tightly wrapped, for 2 to 3 weeks.

Exchanges

1 Fruit

Calories 66
Total Fat 0 g
Saturated Fat 0 g
Calories from Fat 3
Cholesterol 0 mg
Sodium 1 mg
Carbohydrate 17 g
Dietary Fiber 2 g
Sugars 11 g
Protein 1 g

Microwave Wonders

For years I thought I didn't need a microwave. Then I finally got one and realized how useful it was for getting hot food on the table in a hurry. The recipes in this chapter, like Apple Spread, Sweet Potatoes Supreme, and Tangy Mustard Sauce, are designed exclusively for the microwave. In addition, there are others in the book, like the Apple Crisp, that use the microwave for part of the cooking process.

The recipes were all designed in my microwave, which is a high-powered model (900 watts) with a turntable. If your unit has less (or more) power, you may have to adjust the microwaving time slightly. Also, if you do not have a turntable, stop and turn the container at least once during microwaving.

Also, remember that casserole and bowl sizes will make a difference in microwave cooking time. If you use a larger dish than the one specified, you may also have to cook the food longer. I often use a glass measuring cup for microwave cooking because I like the convenience of the handle. Although some people use plastic wrap to cover food being microwaved, I prefer wax paper, since I'm less likely to get burned by escaping steam. Also, when plastic wrap comes in contact with microwaved food, molecules of plastic are left on the surface of the food.

Homemade Pear Spread

Preparation Time: 7 minutes

Serves 16

Serving Size: 1 Tbsp

With a microwave and a food processor fitted with a circular shredder blade, you can make this tasty spread in a snap. Because it's very low in sugar, it makes a great substitute for jam or jelly. Be sure to cook only until the pears are softened and not runny.

1 1/2 cups (about 2 medium) grated or shredded, peeled fresh pear

2 tsp sugar

Scant 1/4 tsp ginger

1/2 tsp vanilla extract

1. In a 2-cup measure or similar small microwave-safe bowl, combine the pear, sugar, and ginger. Stir to mix well.
2. Cover with wax paper and microwave on high power for 2 minutes. Stir. Uncover and microwave an additional 1 to 2 minutes on high power or until the pears are just soft. Stir in vanilla.
3. Serve warm or cover and refrigerate. The spread will keep in the refrigerator for 2 weeks.

Exchanges

Free

Calories 13

Total Fat 0 g

Saturated Fat 0 g

Calories from Fat 1

Cholesterol 0 mg

Sodium 0 mg

Carbohydrate 3 g

Dietary Fiber 0 g

Sugars 3 g

Protein 0 g

Preparation Time:
10 minutes

Serves 16

Serving Size:
1 Tbsp

Homemade Apple Spread

Here's an easy apple spread I use as a topping for bagels or toast. It's mostly fruit, which makes it healthier than jam or even naturally sweetened commercial spreads. I make it with unpeeled apples, but you could peel them if you prefer.

2 cups (about 2 medium) grated or shredded sweet apples

2 Tbsp water

1 Tbsp sugar

1/4 tsp cinnamon

1. After shredding the apples, remove any large pieces of peel. In a 4-cup measure or similar medium microwave-safe bowl, combine the apples, water, sugar, and cinnamon. Stir to mix well.
2. Cover with wax paper and microwave on high power for 2 minutes. Stir. Re-cover and microwave an additional 2 minutes. Stir, recover, and microwave an additional minute, or until the apples are very soft and most of the water has been absorbed.
3. Serve warm, or cover and refrigerate. The spread will keep in the refrigerator for up to 2 weeks.

Exchanges

Free

Calories 13

Total Fat 0 g

Saturated Fat 0 g

Calories from Fat 1

Cholesterol 0 mg

Sodium 0 mg

Carbohydrate 3 g

Dietary Fiber 0 g

Sugars 3 g

Protein 0 g

Tangy Mustard Sauce

Preparation Time: 6 minutes

Serves 8

Serving Size: 1 Tbsp

This flavorful sauce tastes great as a sandwich spread in place of mayonnaise and mustard, mixed with turkey breast meat for a quick turkey salad, or on cooked vegetables, such as cauliflower or carrots.

1 Tbsp packed brown sugar
1 tsp dry mustard
1 Tbsp cider vinegar
1 Tbsp hot water
1/4 cup fat-free sour cream
2 Tbsp reduced-fat mayonnaise

1. In a small microwave-safe bowl, combine the sugar and mustard. Stir to mix well. Stir in the vinegar and water. Cover with wax paper and microwave on high power for 1 minute, or until the flavors are well-blended.
2. Stir and cool slightly. Whisk in the sour cream and mayonnaise. Serve immediately, or cover and refrigerate several hours before serving. The sauce will keep in the refrigerator 4 to 5 days. Stir before serving.

Exchanges

1 Polyunsaturated Fat

Calories 26
Total Fat 1 g
Saturated Fat 0 g
Calories from Fat 10
Cholesterol 2 mg
Sodium 38 mg
Carbohydrate 3 g
Dietary Fiber 0 g
Sugars 3 g
Protein 1 g

Preparation Time:
3 minutes

Serves 2

Serving Size:
1 sweet potato half

Sweet Potatoes Supreme

Sweet potatoes make a great snack. They're high in beta-carotene and fiber. And they microwave beautifully—which means you can fix them in a jiffy.

1 medium sweet potato
2 Tbsp orange or pineapple juice
1/8 tsp ginger
2 Tbsp raisins or other dried fruit bits
2 tsp reduced-fat margarine

1. Pierce the sweet potato with a fork and microwave on high power for 6 to 7 minutes or until tender. Meanwhile, in a 1-cup measure or similar small microwave-safe bowl, stir together the juice and ginger until well mixed. Stir in the raisins.
2. When the sweet potato is tender, remove it from the microwave. Then cover the juice mixture with wax paper and microwave it for 45 seconds to 1 minute on high power, or until heated through.
3. Meanwhile, cut the sweet potato in half and place on two plates. Mash the margarine into the flesh of each half with a fork. Pour the juice mixture over the sweet potato halves, mashing it into the flesh. Serve immediately.

Exchanges
1 1/2 Starch
1/2 Fruit

Calories 138
Total Fat 2 g
Saturated Fat 0 g
Calories from Fat 15
Cholesterol 0 mg
Sodium 40 mg
Carbohydrate 30 g
Dietary Fiber 3 g
Sugars 17 g
Protein 2 g

Con Queso Bean Dip

Keep this piquant Tex-Mex-style dip warm on a hot plate, or return it to the microwave briefly to rewarm it.

1 15 1/2-oz can low-sodium or regular light red kidney beans, rinsed and well drained

3/4 cup mild or medium salsa

1 tsp chili powder

1 tsp cumin

1/8 tsp salt, or to taste (optional)

1 cup shredded reduced-fat Cheddar cheese

1/2 cup fat-free sour cream

2 Tbsp chopped chives or green onions

1. In a 1-quart microwave-safe casserole, mash the beans with a fork. Stir in the salsa, chili powder, cumin, and salt (if desired). Stir to mix well. Stir in the cheese.
2. Cover with the casserole lid, and microwave on high power for 3 to 4 minutes until heated through. Remove from microwave. Stir to mix in the melted cheese. Spread the sour cream on top. Sprinkle with the chives.
3. Serve warm with fat-free tortilla chips. Cover and refrigerate leftovers, which will keep 3 to 4 days.

Preparation Time: 10 minutes

Serves 20

Serving Size: 2 Tbsp

Exchanges

1/2 Starch

Calories 44

Total Fat 1 g

Saturated Fat 1 g

Calories from Fat 12

Cholesterol 4 mg

Sodium 86 mg

Carbohydrate 5 g

Dietary Fiber 1 g

Sugars 1 g

Protein 3 g

Preparation Time:
9 minutes

Serves 6

Serving Size:
1/2 cup

Exchanges

1 Starch

1 Vegetable

Calories 109

Total Fat 2 g

Saturated Fat 0 g

Calories from Fat 15

Cholesterol 0 mg

Sodium 372 mg

Carbohydrate 19 g

Dietary Fiber 3 g

Sugars 3 g

Protein 3 g

Stuffing Pronto

Stuffing for a snack? Sure—if you love it as much as I do. This version, which features a variety of chopped vegetables, is so quick I can indulge myself any time I like. Check package labels to find a stuffing mix that's low in fat and salt.

1 small onion, chopped

1 large celery stalk, diced

1 cup diced cauliflower florets

5 or 6 baby carrots, thinly sliced

1/2 cup fat-free, low-sodium or regular chicken broth

2 Tbsp reduced-fat margarine

1/2 tsp poultry seasoning

Scant 1/4 tsp salt, or to taste (optional)

Dash black pepper

2 cups seasoned commercial crumb-style stuffing

1. In a medium microwave-safe bowl, combine all ingredients except the stuffing and stir to mix well. Cover with wax paper and microwave on high power for 4 to 5 minutes until the vegetables are tender, stopping and stirring the vegetables once during microwaving.
2. Remove the bowl from the microwave and stir in the stuffing mix until well combined. Cover and microwave an additional 2 minutes on high power, stirring once. Serve warm. Leftovers can be stored in the refrigerator for 3 to 4 days.

Fruit Stuffing Pronto

Here's a quick and tasty variation on the stuffing theme, with apples and cranberries as well as vegetables.

1 small onion, chopped
1 medium celery stalk, diced
1 medium apple, cored and chopped
1/2 cup dried cranberries or raisins (or a mixture of the two)
1/2 cup fat-free, low-sodium or regular chicken broth
2 Tbsp reduced-fat margarine
Scant 1/4 tsp salt, or to taste (optional)
Dash black pepper
1/2 tsp poultry seasoning
2 cups seasoned commercial crumb-style stuffing

1. In a medium microwave-safe bowl, combine the onion, celery, apple, cranberries, broth, margarine, salt (if desired), and pepper. Stir to mix well. Cover with wax paper and microwave on high power for 4 to 5 minutes until the onion is tender, stopping and stirring the mixture once during microwaving.
2. Remove the bowl from the microwave and stir in the poultry seasoning. Then stir in the stuffing mix until well combined. Cover and microwave an additional 2 minutes on high power, stopping and stirring once during microwaving.
3. Leftover stuffing will keep in the refrigerator 2 to 3 days.

Preparation Time: 9 minutes

Serves 6

Serving Size: 1/2 cup

Exchanges

1 Starch

1 Fruit

Calories 145

Total Fat 2 g

Saturated Fat 0 g

Calories from Fat 15

Cholesterol 0 mg

Sodium 356 mg

Carbohydrate 28 g

Dietary Fiber 3 g

Sugars 12 g

Protein 3 g

Preparation Time:
15 minutes

Serves 8

Serving Size:
1 piece

Exchanges

1 1/2 Carbohydrate

Calories 117

Total Fat 2 g

Saturated Fat 0 g

Calories from Fat 19

Cholesterol 0 mg

Sodium 101 mg

Carbohydrate 22 g

Dietary Fiber 1 g

Sugars 11 g

Protein 3 g

Apple Scone Cake

Apples add flavor and texture to this quick and easy snack cake.

3 Tbsp reduced-fat tubstyle margarine (4.5 g fat/T)

1 tsp vanilla extract

3 Tbsp sugar

2 large egg whites

3/4 cup all-purpose white flour

1/4 cup oat bran

1 tsp baking powder

1/4 tsp cinnamon

1/8 tsp salt (optional)

1/4 cup low-fat buttermilk

1 large apple, cored, peeled, and thinly sliced

1 1/2 Tbsp sugar

1/4 tsp cinnamon

1. Spray an 8-inch round and at least 2-inch deep (or similar) microwave-safe glass dish with nonstick spray coating. Set aside. In a large mixing bowl with an electric mixer on medium speed, beat together the margarine, vanilla, and sugar. Beat in the egg whites.
2. In a separate medium bowl, stir together the flour, oat bran, baking powder, cinnamon, and salt (if desired). Add the flour mixture and the buttermilk to the margarine mixture, beating until blended. Stir the apple into the batter.
3. Pour the batter into the prepared dish. Rap the dish against the counter top to remove any large

air bubbles. Cover with wax paper, and microwave on 70 percent power for 5 1/2 to 7 1/2 minutes, or until the cake top is just slightly soft when lightly pressed.

4. Mix together the sugar and cinnamon and sprinkle the mixture over the cake. Replace the wax paper and microwave for 1 to 1 1/2 minutes on high power until the sugar has melted and the cake springs back when pressed. Let stand for 5 minutes before serving.

Preparation Time:
15 minutes

Serves 8

Serving Size:
1 piece

Exchanges

1 1/2 Carbohydrate

1/2 Monounsaturated Fat

Calories 128

Total Fat 4 g

Saturated Fat 0 g

Calories from Fat 32

Cholesterol 0 mg

Sodium 102 mg

Carbohydrate 21 g

Dietary Fiber 1 g

Sugars 10 g

Protein 3 g

Honey-Almond Scone Cake

Quick, easy, and full of flavor, this microwave dessert gets extra fiber from oat bran.

3 Tbsp reduced-fat tubstyle margarine (4.5 g fat/T)

1 tsp almond extract

3 Tbsp sugar

2 large egg whites

3/4 cup all-purpose white flour

1/4 cup oat bran

1 tsp baking powder

1/8 tsp salt (optional)

1/4 cup low-fat buttermilk

2 Tbsp mild or strong-flavored honey

1/4 tsp almond extract

3 Tbsp unblanched sliced almonds

1. Spray an 8-inch round and at least 2-inch deep (or similar) microwave-safe glass dish with nonstick spray coating. Set aside. In a large mixing bowl with an electric mixer on medium speed, beat together the margarine, almond extract, and sugar. Beat in the egg whites.
2. In a separate medium bowl, stir together the flour, oat bran, baking powder, and salt (if desired). Add the flour mixture and the buttermilk to the margarine mixture, beating until blended.
3. Pour the batter into the prepared dish. Cover with wax paper and microwave on 70 percent

power for 6 to 8 minutes, or until the cake top springs back when lightly pressed and a toothpick inserted in the center comes out clean. Remove the cake to a wire rack.

4. Mix together the honey and almond extract. With the back of a spoon, spread the mixture over the top of the warm cake. Sprinkle with the almonds. Let stand for 5 minutes before serving.

Preparation Time: 18 minutes

Serves 6

Serving Size: 1/2 cup

Apple Betty

This is one of my favorite old recipes—updated and made a lot healthier. If you want to use very fresh bread, cut slices into cubes and let them dry out on the cutting board for 30 to 40 minutes before using them.

4 cups peeled, diced Red Delicious apples

3 cups 1/4- to 1/2-inch whole-wheat bread cubes

2 Tbsp packed brown sugar

2 Tbsp reduced-fat tubstyle margarine (4.5 g fat/T)

1/2 tsp cinnamon

2 Tbsp hot water

1. Spread half the apples and bread cubes in the bottom of a nonstick 2-quart or similar microwave-safe casserole. Sprinkle with half the brown sugar. Dot with half of the margarine and sprinkle with half of the cinnamon.
2. Repeat with the remaining apples, bread cubes, brown sugar, margarine, and cinnamon. Stir to distribute the ingredients evenly. Pour the water evenly over the top.
3. Cover the casserole with wax paper. Microwave on high power for 6 to 7 minutes. Uncover and stir. Microwave uncovered on high power an additional 2 to 3 minutes, or until the apples are cooked through. The top will not be browned.
4. Serve warm. Top with a small dollop of fat-free yogurt or ice milk, if desired. Leftovers will keep, covered, at room temperature, for 2 days.

Exchanges

1 1/2 Carbohydrate

1/2 Monounsaturated Fat

Calories 119

Total Fat 2 g

Saturated Fat 0 g

Calories from Fat 22

Cholesterol 0 mg

Sodium 106 mg

Carbohydrate 25 g

Dietary Fiber 3 g

Sugars 17 g

Protein 2 g

Delectable Desserts

It used to be that sugar was forbidden in the meal plans of people with diabetes. But as researchers learned more about the chemistry of food, they came to the conclusion that sugars are not a special class of foods. They are just simple carbohydrates, and no more harmful than complex carbohydrates like potatoes, pasta, and bread. And it is the total amount of carbohydrates eaten that affects blood glucose levels, not where they come from.

That means you can include some foods with sugar in your meal plan, as long as you account for the carbohydrate total in the rest of your daily food choices. Although you can't go overboard on sugar, you can substitute sugar for other foods that have approximately the same number of total carbohydrates. If you want to eat a serving of Apple Crisp or the Pumpkin Spice Muffins in this chapter, have them instead of a bread roll or a portion of pasta.

Not only have I kept sugar to a minimum in these recipes, I've also cut the fat and calories, so you can enjoy a serving of these treats without guilt. And I've also taken advantage of the natural sugars in fruits, which are high in the vitamins, minerals, and fiber that should be included in your diet every day.

While many of the recipes in this chapter are made from scratch, some do take advantage of some convenience foods available in your grocery store. Several, like the Apricot Kuchen and Pecan Buns, use refrigerator buttermilk biscuits. And you'll find elegant Pastry Cups and Cherry Tarts made from phyllo dough, which you can purchase in the frozen food section of most supermarkets.

By the way, you will find additional sweet treats in two other chapters: Just For Kids and Microwave Wonders.

Preparation Time: 6 minutes

Serves 5

Serving Size: 1/3 cup

Vanilla Custard

This wonderfully creamy custard tastes great by itself or with fruit. It's also used in the Cherry Tarts on p. 173.

1 egg yolk

1 3/4 cups low-fat (1%) milk

3 Tbsp sugar

2 Tbsp cornstarch

1 tsp butter or regular margarine

3/4 tsp vanilla extract

1. In a 2-cup glass measure or similar microwave-safe bowl, beat together the egg and milk with a fork or wire whisk. Cover with wax paper and microwave on high power for 2 to 2 1/2 minutes, stopping and stirring three times, until the mixture is hot but not boiling.
2. In the top of a double boiler, mix together the sugar and cornstarch. Gradually whisk or stir in the heated milk mixture, stirring vigorously and scraping the pan bottom until smooth. Cook over boiling water, stirring vigorously, for 3 to 4 minutes, or until the mixture thickens.
3. Remove from heat. Stir in the butter and vanilla. Cool slightly. Serve warm, or cover and refrigerate 3 to 4 hours or up to 48 hours.

Exchanges

1 Carbohydrate

1/2 Saturated Fat

Calories 95

Total Fat 3 g

Saturated Fat 2 g

Calories from Fat 24

Cholesterol 48 mg

Sodium 53 mg

Carbohydrate 15 g

Dietary Fiber 0 g

Sugars 11 g

Protein 3 g

Pastry Cups

Preparation Time: 15 minutes

Serves 12

Serving Size: 1 cup

Virtually fat-free, these elegant but easy phyllo cups make the perfect shell for a variety of desserts. Fill them with cut fruit, or make the rich-tasting Cherry Tarts on p. 173.
For additional information on phyllo, see the note on Spanakopita Bake, p. 90.

3 large phyllo sheets, thawed
Butter-flavored nonstick spray coating

1. Spray a 12-cup standard muffin tin with butter-flavored nonstick spray coating. Set aside. Preheat the oven to 400 degrees.
2. Lay the phyllo on a large plastic cutting board or other flat surface. Using sharp scissors or a sharp knife, cut each pastry sheet into 4- to 4 1/2-inch squares. Stack the squares, and keep them covered with wax paper until you are ready for them.
3. Spray 3 squares with butter-flavored nonstick spray coating. Place the squares on top of each other, rotating them slightly so that the corners are facing in different directions. Gently press the squares into a muffin cup, making a basket. Repeat the process to make 12 cups.
4. Bake on the center oven rack for 4 to 5 minutes or until the edges of the cups begin to crisp. Cups can be cooled slightly and filled with desired filling. Or they can be cooled, covered with plastic wrap, and stored in the refrigerator for 3 to 4 days before filling. They should not be filled until 2 to 3 hours before serving.

Exchange

Free

Calories 18
Total Fat 0 g
Saturated Fat 0 g
Calories from Fat 1
Cholesterol 0 mg
Sodium 30 mg
Carbohydrate 4 g
Dietary Fiber 0 g
Sugars 0 g
Protein 1 g

Pear Cups

Preparation Time: 10 minutes

Serves 6

Serving Size: 1 cup

With phyllo dough, you can quickly make these easy and festive baked pear tarts.

Butter-flavored nonstick spray coating

1 1/2 large phyllo sheets, thawed

6 juice-packed canned pear halves

2 tsp sugar

1/8 tsp cinnamon

1. Spray a 6-cup standard muffin tin with butter-flavored nonstick spray coating. Preheat the oven to 400 degrees.
2. Lay the phyllo on a large plastic cutting board or other flat surface. Using sharp scissors or a sharp knife, cut each pastry sheet into six 4- to 4 1/2-inch squares. Keep the squares covered with wax paper until you are ready for them.
3. Spray 3 squares with butter-flavored nonstick spray coating. Place the squares on top of each other, rotating them slightly so that the corners are facing in different directions. Gently press the squares into a muffin cup, making a basket. Repeat the process to make 6 cups.
4. Lay a pear half, cut side up, in each cup. Mix together the sugar and cinnamon. Sprinkle each pear lightly with the mixture, dividing evenly. Bake on the center oven rack for 5 to 6 minutes or until the edges of the cups begin to crisp. Cool slightly on a wire rack. Serve warm. Leftover cups can be covered and refrigerated for 3 to 4 days. They can be served chilled.

Exchanges

1 Fruit

Calories 54

Total Fat 0 g

Saturated Fat 0 g

Calories from Fat 1

Cholesterol 0 mg

Sodium 33 mg

Carbohydrate 13 g

Dietary Fiber 1 g

Sugars 7 g

Protein 1 g

Cherry Tarts

Preparation Time: 20 minutes

Serves 12

Serving Size: 1 tart

For an elegant end to a special meal—or a wonderful tea-time treat—try this sumptuous cherry tart.

1 20-oz can lite cherry pie filling

1/4 tsp cinnamon

1 recipe Pastry Cups (p. 171)

1 recipe Vanilla Custard (p. 170)

1. Stir together the cherry pie filling and cinnamon. Set aside.
2. Set each pastry shell on a serving plate. Spoon 2 Tbsp of custard into each. Spoon 2 1/2 Tbsp of cherry pie filling over custard.
3. Serve at once. Or fill shells up to 2 hours before needed, and refrigerate.

Exchanges

1 Carbohydrate

Calories 91

Total Fat 1 g

Saturated Fat 1 g

Calories from Fat 12

Cholesterol 20 mg

Sodium 60 mg

Carbohydrate 18 g

Dietary Fiber 1 g

Sugars 12 g

Protein 2 g

Preparation Time:
20 minutes

Serves 8

Serving Size:
1 piece

Peach Cobbler

Here's a wonderful late summer combination—peaches with a biscuit topping. Starting the fruit in the microwave gives the peaches a well-baked taste and texture.

3 Tbsp sugar

2 Tbsp white flour

1/4 tsp cinnamon

4 cups peeled and sliced ripe peaches

1 cup white flour

1 Tbsp sugar

1 1/2 tsp baking powder

1/8 tsp salt

3 Tbsp reduced-fat margarine

1/2 cup low-fat (1%) milk

1. Preheat the oven to 400 degrees. In a microwave-safe, oven-proof 2-quart casserole, combine the sugar, flour, and cinnamon. Add the peaches, and stir until all of the flour mixture coats the peaches. Cover with the casserole lid, and microwave on high power for about 4 minutes, stirring twice, or until the peaches have softened and are surrounded by a thickened sauce. Reserve the peaches in the microwave.
2. In a medium bowl, combine the flour, sugar, baking powder, and salt. Stir to mix well. With a fork or fingers, blend in margarine until completely incorporated. Stir in the milk. The batter will be slightly soupy.

Exchanges

2 Carbohydrate

Calories 140

Total Fat 2 g

Saturated Fat 0 g

Calories from Fat 18

Cholesterol 1 mg

Sodium 146 mg

Carbohydrate 28 g

Dietary Fiber 2 g

Sugars 13 g

Protein 3 g

3. Remove the casserole from the microwave. Divide the dough into 8 portions (about 2 Tbsp each). Drop the dough onto the hot peach mixture. Bake in the preheated oven 18 to 25 minutes or until the filling is bubbly and topping is set and beginning to brown. Cool 5 minutes before serving.
4. The cobbler is best served warm. It will keep, covered, at room temperature for about 2 days.

Preparation Time: 6 minutes

Serves 8

Serving Size: 1 piece

Exchanges

1 1/2 Carbohydrate

Calories 98

Total Fat 1 g

Saturated Fat 0 g

Calories from Fat 10

Cholesterol 0 mg

Sodium 232 mg

Carbohydrate 21 g

Dietary Fiber 1 g

Sugars 9 g

Protein 2 g

Apricot Kuchen

Here's a delicious, practically instant apricot kuchen, with a crust made from refrigerator buttermilk biscuits. When measuring out the apricot preserves, use plastic measuring spoons so they can go in the microwave.

1 15-oz can juice-packed apricot halves

1 7 1/2-oz package reduced-fat refrigerator buttermilk biscuits

1 tsp reduced-fat tubstyle margarine (4.5 g fat/T)

1 1/2 Tbsp apricot preserves

1 Tbsp sugar

1. Preheat the oven to 450 degrees. Spray a 9-inch pie plate with nonstick spray coating. Set aside. Drain the apricots well in a colander. Blot them dry with paper towels.
2. Open the biscuit carton and separate the biscuits. Place them on the pie plate and press and squeeze the inner edges together so that they touch and cover the bottom of the plate. With your finger or the back of a spoon, spread the margarine on the biscuits, dividing it evenly.
3. Lay the measuring spoons of apricot preserves on a plate, and microwave at full power for 10 to 15 seconds to soften. Drizzle the melted preserves over the margarine, and spread it evenly with the back of the spoon.
4. Arrange the apricot halves, cut side down, in an attractive pattern over the biscuits. Sprinkle the kuchen top evenly with the sugar.

5. Bake in the center of the oven for 11 to 13 minutes or until the edges of the biscuits are well browned and the liquid at the edge of the plate is bubbly. Serve hot. Leftover kuchen will keep for 1 to 2 days at room temperature, if tightly wrapped.

Preparation Time:
20 minutes

Serves 15

Serving Size:
1 piece

Exchanges

1 1/2 Carbohydrate

1/2 Saturated Fat

Calories 150

Total Fat 3 g

Saturated Fat 2 g

Calories from Fat 29

Cholesterol 37 mg

Sodium 176 mg

Carbohydrate 22 g

Dietary Fiber 1 g

Sugars 12 g

Protein 7 g

Noodle Pudding

Serve this tasty pudding to a crowd of hungry snackers.

6 cups uncooked medium-sized reduced-fat egg noodles

5 oz Neufchâtel cheese, at room temperature

1/4 cup sugar

2 large eggs plus 3 large egg whites

1 cup reduced-fat cottage cheese

3/4 cup plain fat-free yogurt

2 1/2 tsp vanilla extract

Generous 1/4 tsp salt

1 8-oz can crushed juice-packed pineapple, well drained

1/2 cup dried cranberries or raisins

1 1/2 Tbsp sugar

1/4 tsp cinnamon

1. Preheat the oven to 375 degrees. Spray a 9- by 13-inch baking pan with nonstick spray coating and set aside. Cook noodles according to package directions. Drain well.
2. Meanwhile, in a large mixer bowl, combine the cream cheese and 1/4 cup sugar. Beat on medium speed until well combined and smooth. Add the eggs and egg whites, cottage cheese, yogurt, vanilla, and salt. Beat on medium speed. When partially combined, increase speed to high, and beat until well combined.

3. Stir in the pineapple and dried cranberries. Stir in the noodles. Turn out into the prepared dish, and spread evenly, using the back of a large spoon. Stir together the sugar and cinnamon. Sprinkle the mixture evenly over the noodle mixture.
4. Bake for 35 to 40 minutes until just set and a toothpick inserted in the center comes out clean. Do not overbake.

Preparation Time: 20 minutes

Serves 12

Serving Size: 1 muffin

Exchanges

1 1/2 Carbohydrate

1 Monounsaturated Fat

Calories 162

Total Fat 5 g

Saturated Fat 0 g

Calories from Fat 47

Cholesterol 1 mg

Sodium 116 mg

Carbohydrate 26 g

Dietary Fiber 1 g

Sugars 9 g

Protein 4 g

Cranberry-Orange Muffins

Here's a fruit muffin you can enjoy as a snack or for breakfast

1/4 cup dried cranberries
1/3 cup orange juice
1 1/3 cups all-purpose white flour
3/4 cup whole-wheat flour
1/3 cup sugar
2 1/2 tsp baking powder
1/8 tsp ginger
1/8 tsp salt
1 cup low-fat (1%) milk
1 large egg white
1/4 cup canola or safflower oil
2 tsp vanilla extract

1. Preheat the oven to 425 degrees. Coat a 12-cup standard muffin tin with nonstick spray coating and set aside. Chop the cranberries. In a 2-cup microwave-safe measure, combine the cranberries and orange juice. Cover with wax paper and microwave on high power for 1 minute, or until the cranberries are softened. Set aside.
2. In a large bowl, stir together the white flour, whole-wheat flour, sugar, baking powder, ginger, and salt. Add the milk, egg white, oil, and vanilla to the measuring cup with the cranberry-orange mixture. Stir with a fork until well mixed.
3. Gently stir the cranberry mixture into the dry ingredients until just incorporated. Do not

overmix. Divide the batter evenly among the muffin cups. (They will be almost full.) Bake on the center oven rack for 15 to 18 minutes, or until the muffins are lightly browned and a toothpick inserted in the center of one comes out clean. Transfer the pan to a wire rack, and let it stand for 5 minutes before removing the muffins.

4. The muffins will keep for 1 to 2 days at room temperature if tightly wrapped. Freeze for longer storage.

Preparation Time: 20 minutes

Serves 12

Serving Size: 1 muffin

Exchanges

2 Carbohydrate

1/2 Monounsaturated Fat

Calories 158

Total Fat 4 g

Saturated Fat 0 g

Calories from Fat 36

Cholesterol 1 mg

Sodium 146 mg

Carbohydrate 28 g

Dietary Fiber 2 g

Sugars 13 g

Protein 3 g

Pineapple-Carrot Muffins

I love the combination of tastes and textures in these muffins, which make a great snack or a quick breakfast. You can make them with clover honey, but they're more flavorful with a stronger-flavored honey, such as locust or buckwheat.

1 cup all-purpose white flour
3/4 cup whole-wheat flour
3 Tbsp sugar
2 tsp baking powder
1/2 tsp baking soda
1 tsp cinnamon
1/8 tsp cloves
1/8 tsp salt (optional)
Scant 1 cup low-fat buttermilk
3 Tbsp canola or olive oil
1 large egg white
2 Tbsp mild or strong-flavored honey
1 8-oz can juice-packed crushed pineapple, well drained
1 medium carrot, grated or shredded
1/2 cup dark seedless raisins

1. Preheat the oven to 400 degrees. Coat a 12-cup standard muffin tin with nonstick spray coating and set aside. In a medium bowl, combine the flours, sugar, baking powder, baking soda, cinnamon, cloves, and salt (if desired), and stir to mix well.

2. In a small bowl, blend the buttermilk, oil, egg white, and honey with a fork. Add to the dry mixture, and stir to incorporate, but do not overmix. Stir in the pineapple, shredded carrot, and raisins. Divide the batter evenly among muffin tin cups. (Cups will be almost full.)
3. Bake for 22 to 25 minutes or until the tops of the muffins are browned. The muffins taste best warm and fresh but will keep for 1 to 2 days at room temperature if tightly wrapped. Freeze for longer storage.

Preparation Time: 15 minutes

Serves 12

Serving Size: 1 muffin

Pumpkin Spice Muffins

If you like gingerbread, you'll love these muffins!

1 cup oat bran

1 cup all-purpose white flour

1/4 cup sugar

1 tsp baking powder

1/2 tsp baking soda

1 tsp pumpkin pie spice

1/8 tsp salt

1/4 cup liquid egg substitute

1/2 cup low-fat buttermilk

1/2 cup canned solid-pack pumpkin (not pumpkin pie filling)

3 Tbsp canola or corn oil

2 Tbsp dark molasses

3/4 cup dark or light raisins

1. Preheat the oven to 400 degrees. Coat a 12-cup standard muffin tin with nonstick spray coating and set aside. In a large bowl, combine the oat bran, flour, sugar, baking powder, baking soda, pumpkin pie spice, and salt. Stir to mix well.
2. Add the egg substitute, buttermilk, pumpkin, oil, and molasses. Stir until just mixed. Stir in the raisins. Spoon the batter into the muffin tin cups. Bake for 16 to 19 minutes, or until the muffins are springy to the touch and lightly browned.
3. Cool for 2 to 3 minutes and remove. These muffins taste great warm and can also be stored at room temperature in an airtight container for 2 to 3 days. Freeze for longer storage.

Exchanges

2 Carbohydrate

1/2 Monounsaturated Fat

Calories 159

Total Fat 4 g

Saturated Fat 0 g

Calories from Fat 39

Cholesterol 0 mg

Sodium 131 mg

Carbohydrate 27 g

Dietary Fiber 2 g

Sugars 13 g

Protein 4 g

Apple Crisp

Preparation Time: 18 minutes

Serves 8

Serving Size: 1/2 cup

If you like cooked apples, you'll love the taste of this easy crisp. Starting the apples in the microwave gives them a well-baked texture.

6 cups thinly sliced, peeled, tart apples
2 Tbsp all-purpose white flour
1 Tbsp sugar
1/2 tsp cinnamon
1/2 cup quick-cooking rolled oats
1/4 cup all-purpose white flour
3 Tbsp packed light brown sugar
2 Tbsp reduced-fat tubstyle margarine (4.5 g fat/T)

1. Preheat the oven to 400 degrees. In a large bowl, combine the apples, 2 Tbsp flour, sugar, and cinnamon. Stir to mix well. Transfer the mixture to a nonstick spray-coated 10-inch microwave-safe pie plate. Cover with wax paper, and microwave on high power for about 4 minutes or until the apples are partially cooked.
2. Meanwhile, for the topping, in a medium bowl, combine the oats, flour, and brown sugar. Mix well with a fork or fingers. Blend in margarine with a fork or fingers until completely incorporated. Distribute the topping over the apples.
3. Bake in the oven for 22 to 28 minutes or until the apples are tender when pierced with a fork and the filling is bubbly. Leftovers can be stored covered, at room temperature, for 2 to 3 days.

Exchanges

2 Carbohydrate

Calories 144
Total Fat 2 g
Saturated Fat 0 g
Calories from Fat 17
Cholesterol 0 mg
Sodium 25 mg
Carbohydrate 32 g
Dietary Fiber 3 g
Sugars 22 g
Protein 2 g

Preparation Time:
12 minutes

Serves 12

Serving Size:
1 muffin

Exchanges

1 1/2 Carbohydrate

Calories 115

Total Fat 2 g

Saturated Fat 0 g

Calories from Fat 18

Cholesterol 1 mg

Sodium 173 mg

Carbohydrate 21 g

Dietary Fiber 2 g

Sugars 8 g

Protein 4 g

Blueberry Muffins

These are packed with flavor and fiber!

1 cup all-purpose white flour

1 cup oat bran

1/3 cup sugar

1 1/2 tsp baking powder

1/2 tsp baking soda

1/2 tsp lemon zest

1/8 tsp salt

3 Tbsp reduced-fat tubstyle margarine (4.5 g fat/T)

1 large egg white

1 cup low-fat buttermilk

1/8 tsp lemon extract

1 1/4 cups fresh or dry-packed (unsweetened) frozen blueberries

1. Preheat the oven to 400 degrees. Spray a 12-cup standard muffin tin with nonstick spray coating and set aside. In a large bowl, combine the flour, oat bran, sugar, baking powder, baking soda, lemon zest, and salt and stir to mix well.
2. With a pastry cutter or two forks, blend in the margarine until it is completely incorporated and the mixture resembles coarse meal. Add the egg white, buttermilk, and lemon extract. Stir until just mixed. Gently stir in the blueberries.
3. Divide the batter evenly among the muffin cups. Bake for 16 to 20 minutes or until nicely browned. Remove the muffins immediately to a wire rack. Serve warm. Muffins will keep at room temperature for 2 to 3 days if tightly wrapped.

Cinnamon Biscuits

Preparation Time: 6 minutes

Serves 6

Serving Size: 1 biscuit

A little sugar and margarine go a long way on these fun and easy-to-make cinnamon biscuits. Note that I've used a small package of biscuits for this very quick but very tasty recipe.

1 1/2 tsp sugar

Generous pinch cinnamon

1 4 1/2-oz package reduced-fat refrigerator buttermilk biscuits

1 tsp reduced-fat tubstyle margarine (4.5 g fat/T)

1. Preheat the oven to 450 degrees. Spray a small baking sheet with nonstick spray coating and set aside.
2. In a custard cup, mix together the sugar and cinnamon. Open the biscuit carton, and separate the biscuits. Set the biscuits on the baking sheet.
3. With your finger or the back of a spoon, brush the top of each biscuit with margarine, dividing it evenly. Sprinkle the cinnamon-sugar mixture over the top of each biscuit, dividing it evenly.
4. Bake in the center of the oven for 8 to 10 minutes or until golden. Serve hot.

Exchanges

1/2 Starch

Calories 56

Total Fat 1 g

Saturated Fat 0 g

Calories from Fat 9

Cholesterol 0 mg

Sodium 185 mg

Carbohydrate 11 g

Dietary Fiber 0 g

Sugars 2 g

Protein 1 g

Preparation Time: 4 minutes

Serves 10

Serving Size: 1 bun

Pecan Buns

You won't believe how easy it is to make these rich-tasting pecan buns. You can use mild honey, but one with a stronger taste, such as buckwheat, will add more flavor to the buns.

1 7 1/2-oz package reduced-fat refrigerator buttermilk biscuits

1 tsp reduced-fat tubstyle margarine (4.5 g fat/T)

1 1/2 Tbsp mild or strong-flavored honey

2 Tbsp finely chopped pecans

1. Preheat the oven to 450 degrees. Spray a 9-inch pie plate with nonstick spray coating and set aside.
2. Open the biscuit carton and separate the biscuits. Place them on the pie plate so that they are barely touching.
3. With your finger or the back of a spoon, spread the margarine on the biscuits, dividing it evenly. Pour the honey on the biscuits, dividing it evenly, and spread it to cover the biscuit tops. Sprinkle the biscuits with the pecans.
4. Bake in the center of the oven for 8 to 10 minutes or until golden. Serve hot. Leftover buns will keep at room temperature for 1 to 2 days, if tightly covered. They can be served as is or rewarmed quickly in the microwave or toaster oven.

Exchanges

1 Carbohydrate

Calories 69

Total Fat 2 g

Saturated Fat 0 g

Calories from Fat 15

Cholesterol 0 mg

Sodium 183 mg

Carbohydrate 13 g

Dietary Fiber 0 g

Sugars 4 g

Protein 1 g

Apple-Cranberry Turnovers

Use refrigerator biscuits for a quick dessert!

1 medium apple, peeled, cored, and diced
2 Tbsp dried cranberries
1 Tbsp sugar
1/4 tsp cinnamon
2 Tbsp water
1 7 1/2-oz package reduced-fat refrigerator buttermilk biscuits

1. Preheat the oven to 400 degrees. Spray a baking sheet with nonstick spray coating and set aside.
2. In a 2-cup measure or similar small microwave-safe bowl, combine the apple, cranberries, sugar, and cinnamon. Stir to mix. Stir in the water. Cover with wax paper and microwave on high power for 3 minutes, stopping and stirring once during microwaving. Cool slightly.
3. Working on a nonstick spray-coated surface, flatten each biscuit into a three-inch round. Spoon about 2 tsp of the mixture into the center of the biscuit. Fold the biscuit in half over the filling, making a turnover shape. Seal the edges by pressing closed with fingers, then with the tines of a fork. Lay the biscuits on the prepared baking sheet. Prick the top of each turnover with the fork tines.
4. Bake for 8 to 10 minutes, or until the tops of the biscuits begin to brown. Serve hot. Leftovers will keep for 1 to 2 days, tightly covered, at room temperature.

Preparation Time: 10 minutes

Serves 10

Serving Size: 1 turnover

Exchanges

1 Carbohydrate

Calories 68
Total Fat 1 g
Saturated Fat 0 g
Calories from Fat 7
Cholesterol 0 mg
Sodium 180 mg
Carbohydrate 14 g
Dietary Fiber 1 g
Sugars 5 g
Protein 1 g

More Scrumptious Snacks

These new recipes feature the use of monounsaturated and polyunsaturated fats found in oils, such as canola oil and olive oil, and in nuts. Nuts add great flavor and excellent nutrition to many snacks. Enjoy some crisp Cabbage and Peanut Slaw. Or try the Summer Cheesecake with its crunchy pie crust made of ground pecans.

I like to serve mini-meals, so my snacks are especially hearty and good. These recipes are tasty enough to serve to your favorite guests, and easy enough to make just for yourself. There are plenty of dips to offer at your next party, and some delicious desserts like Marzipan Candy and Red, White, and Blue Fruit Tart.

Red, White, and Green Bean Dip

Beans are a wonderful food, high in flavor and fiber. Serve this dip with whole-wheat pita bread triangles or whole-wheat crackers.

Preparation Time: 12 minutes

Serves 11

Serving Size: 2 Tbsp

1 19-oz can cannellini beans, rinsed and drained
2 1/2 Tbsp extra-virgin olive oil
2 Tbsp chopped parsley leaves
2 Tbsp chopped chives or sliced green onions
1 Tbsp lemon juice
1/2 tsp dried rosemary leaves
1 tsp chopped garlic
1/4 tsp salt, or to taste (optional)
1/8 tsp white pepper
2 Tbsp chopped pimiento

1. In a food processor, combine the beans, oil, parsley, chives, lemon juice, rosemary, garlic, salt (if using), and pepper. Process until smooth. Stir in pimiento.
2. Serve at once or cover and refrigerate until chilled. Dip will keep in the refrigerator 2 to 3 days.

Exchanges

1/2 Starch

1/2 Fat

Calories 73

Total Fat 3 g

Saturated Fat 0 g

Calories from Fat 29

Cholesterol 0 mg

Sodium 89 mg

Carbohydrate 8 g

Dietary Fiber 2 g

Sugars 0 g

Protein 3 g

Preparation Time:
15 minutes

Serves 14

Serving Size:
2 Tbsp

Salsa Bean Dip

This easy Southwestern-style bean dip is high in taste appeal. To get the right texture, you must drain the salsa. The preparation time looks long, but much of this time includes draining the salsa. You can use either mild or medium salsa in the dip. If you use mild and find you'd like it spicier, add a bit of hot sauce.

3/4 cup mild or medium thick and chunky salsa
1 19-oz can cannellini beans, rinsed and drained
1 tsp lemon juice
1 tsp dark chili powder (or to taste)
1 tsp ground cumin
1/8 tsp salt

1. Place the salsa in a sieve over a large bowl. Tap the sieve occasionally to help the salsa drain until the chunky part remains in the sieve, about 3 to 4 minutes. Discard the liquid.
2. In the bowl, mash the beans slightly with a fork.
3. Add the chunky portion of the salsa, lemon juice, chili powder, and cumin. Stir until combined. Transfer to a serving bowl.
4. Serve at once or cover and refrigerate for several hours. Serve with baked corn chips. Leftover dip will keep in the refrigerator for 3 to 4 days.

Exchanges

1/2 Starch

Calories 36
Total Fat 0 g
Saturated Fat 0 g
Calories from Fat 2
Cholesterol 0 mg
Sodium 74 mg
Carbohydrate 7 g
Dietary Fiber 2 g
Sugars 0 g
Protein 2 g

Blue Cheese Spread

Preparation Time: 12 minutes

Serves 32

Serving Size: 2 tsp

Here's a cheese spread with crowd appeal. My guests love the mild blue cheese flavor and the crunch of pecans and celery.

5 oz reduced-fat cream cheese

3 oz fat-free cream cheese

1/2 cup crumbled blue cheese

1 tsp instant minced onion

Dash garlic powder

1 large stalk celery, finely diced

1/4 cup finely chopped pecans

1. In a medium bowl, combine the cream cheeses, blue cheese, onion, and garlic powder.
2. Mash and stir with a fork until mixed. Stir in the celery and pecans. Transfer to a serving bowl. Serve at once or cover with plastic wrap and refrigerate 1 to 2 hours. Cheese spread will keep in the refrigerator for up to a week.

Exchanges

1/2 Fat

Calories 26

Total Fat 2 g

Saturated Fat 1 g

Calories from Fat 19

Cholesterol 5 mg

Sodium 59 mg

Carbohydrate 1 g

Dietary Fiber 0 g

Sugars 0 g

Protein 1 g

Preparation Time: 15 minutes

Serves 8

Serving Size: 3/4 cup

Exchanges

1 Vegetable

1 1/2 Fat

Calories 102

Total Fat 8 g

Saturated Fat 1 g

Calories from Fat 71

Cholesterol 5 mg

Sodium 233 mg

Carbohydrate 6 g

Dietary Fiber 1 g

Sugars 2 g

Protein 3 g

Antipasto

If you like Italian-style antipasto, try this easy version. It's perfect for a company appetizer. Or whip up a batch and keep it in the refrigerator, just for the family. I like the taste of freshly-made dressing with this dish, but if you prefer, you can use low-fat bottled Italian dressing. Rather than using Italian cold cuts, which tend to be quite high in fat, I've substituted cooked lean Canadian bacon.

Dressing:

1/4 cup olive oil, preferably extra virgin

1/2 Tbsp water

2 tsp lemon juice

1 tsp red wine vinegar

1 tsp Italian seasoning

Vegetables and Meat:

1 14 1/2-oz can artichoke heart quarters, well drained

2 cups grape tomatoes

1 coarsely sliced celery stalk

1/2 red pepper, seeded and cut into strips

1/2 yellow pepper, seeded and cut into strips

3 oz cooked lean Canadian bacon, cut into thin strips

1. In a large bowl, combine the oil, water, lemon juice, vinegar, and Italian seasoning. Stir to mix well.
2. Remove any coarse outer leaves from the artichoke hearts. Stir the artichoke hearts, tomatoes, celery, peppers, and Canadian bacon into the dressing, and gently toss to coat.
3. If desired, transfer to a shallow serving dish or platter. Serve at once, or cover and refrigerate up to 24 hours. Antipasto will keep in the refrigerator for 3 to 4 days.

Preparation Time: 15 minutes

Serves 4

Serving Size: 1 cup

Cabbage and Peanut Slaw

In this crunchy coleslaw variation, the peanuts add not only texture, but an interesting flavor.

1/3 cup reduced-fat mayonnaise

1 1/2 Tbsp cider vinegar

1 1/2 Tbsp Splenda

5 cups very thinly sliced green cabbage

2 Tbsp chopped red onion

1/2 cup unsalted or salted peanuts, coarsely chopped

1. In a large bowl, whisk together the mayonnaise, vinegar, and Splenda.
2. Add the cabbage, onion, and peanuts. Stir to mix well. Serve immediately or cover and refrigerate up to 24 hours before serving. Coleslaw will keep in the refrigerator 3 to 4 days.

Exchanges

3 Fat

1 Carbohydrate

Calories 201

Total Fat 16 g

Saturated Fat 3 g

Calories from Fat 144

Cholesterol 7 mg

Sodium 178 mg

Carbohydrate 11 g

Dietary Fiber 4 g

Sugars 4 g

Protein 6 g

Red, White, and Blue Fruit Tart

Preparation Time: 30 minutes

Serves 8

Serving Size: 1/8 tart

I love to serve this dessert for company, although I always hope there will be leftovers for me! I've made the crust of this tart from ground almonds. If you like marzipan, you'll love the taste. I like to use strawberries and blueberries for the topping. But you could substitute peaches or raspberries if you like.

1 Marzipan Crust (see recipe, p. 205)
3 oz reduced-fat cream cheese, at room temperature
1 Tbsp reduced-fat (2%) milk
1 Tbsp Splenda
1 cup washed, hulled, and sliced strawberries
1/2 cup blueberries, washed and picked over

1. Make Marzipan Crust. Set aside.
2. In a small bowl, combine the cream cheese, milk, and Splenda; stir with a soup spoon until uniform. With the back of the spoon, spread the mixture over the prepared crust.
3. Attractively arrange the fruit over the cream cheese mixture. For example, you can make a circle of blueberries at the outer edge of the crust and mound the additional berries in the center of the crust. Then add two rings of sliced strawberries in the remaining space. Refrigerate.
4. When cool, cover with plastic wrap, or serve the tart immediately. The tart can be made up to 12 hours before serving. It will keep in the refrigerator for 2 to 3 days, but the cream cheese layer may start to absorb color from the fruit after 24 hours. Alternatively, you can make the crust the day before, then complete the tart before serving.

Exchanges

3 Fat

1/2 Carbohydrate

Calories 174

Total Fat 13 g

Saturated Fat 2 g

Calories from Fat 120

Cholesterol 8 mg

Sodium 64 mg

Carbohydrate 9 g

Dietary Fiber 4 g

Sugars 4 g

Protein 6 g

Cranberry Orange Tart

Preparation Time: 30 minutes

Serves 6

Serving Size: 1/6 tart

Fresh cranberries give this tart its wonderful tang. Since they are only available in the fall, I buy a lot of them and freeze them for later use. To speed the jelling of the cranberry mixture, you can put the saucepan in the freezer, but check it periodically to make sure the mixture doesn't freeze. The marzipan crust tastes wonderful with the cranberries.

1 Marzipan Crust (see recipe, p. 205)

1 1/3 cups fresh cranberries, washed and picked over

1 cup Splenda

1 cup hot water, divided

1 packet unflavored gelatin

1 tsp vanilla extract

1/2 tsp orange extract

1. Make Marzipan Crust. Set aside.
2. In a food processor, chop the cranberries until finely chopped.
3. Transfer the cranberries to a medium saucepan. Stir in the Splenda and 1/2 cup of the water. Bring to a boil. Reduce the heat and simmer, uncovered, 10 to 15 minutes or until the cranberries are partially cooked.

Exchanges

3 Fat

1 Carbohydrate

Calories 212

Total Fat 15 g

Saturated Fat 0 g

Calories from Fat 132

Cholesterol 0 mg

Sodium 25 mg

Carbohydrate 15 g

Dietary Fiber 5 g

Sugars 8 g

Protein 7 g

4. Meanwhile, stir the gelatin into the remaining hot water until dissolved. While the cranberries are simmering, stir the gelatin mixture into the cranberry mixture. Return to a boil. Reduce the heat and continue to simmer. When cooked, stir in the vanilla and orange extract.
5. Refrigerate the cranberry mixture until partially set, then spread it on the prepared marzipan crust. Refrigerate until set, 1 to 2 hours. After the tart is set, cover with plastic wrap. Tart can be made the day before needed, or make the crust the day before and cover and refrigerate. Leftovers will keep for 3 to 4 days.

Preparation Time: 30 minutes

Serves 9

Serving Size: 1/9 cheesecake

Exchanges

1 Medium-Fat Meat

3 Fat

1 Carbohydrate

Calories 272

Total Fat 21 g

Saturated Fat 9 g

Calories from Fat 187

Cholesterol 45 mg

Sodium 178 mg

Carbohydrate 11 g

Dietary Fiber 1 g

Sugars 7 g

Protein 11 g

New York Cheesecake

Designed for cheesecake lovers, this wonderful New York-style cheesecake is much lower in fat than the traditional version. The crust is made from pecans, but you don't need a lot of them to impart a tasty nutty flavor. Since the crust is made by spreading a layer of pecans on the bottom of the pan, you will need to carefully spoon the cheesecake mixture over them to make sure they remain in place.

3/4 cup very finely ground pecans (1 cup whole pecans)

1 15-oz carton part-skim ricotta cheese

1 cup plain low-fat yogurt

1 cup Splenda

1/2 cup fat-free liquid egg substitute

2 Tbsp white flour

1 Tbsp vanilla extract

Zest (grated rind) of one small lemon

1 8-oz package cream cheese, at room temperature

1. Preheat the oven to 350 degrees.
2. Spray a 10-inch springform pan with nonstick spray.
3. Sprinkle the ground pecans evenly over the pan bottom, patting them into place. The crust layer will be very light and may not entirely cover the bottom of the pan.

4. In a food processor, combine the ricotta, yogurt, Splenda, egg substitute, flour, vanilla, and lemon zest. Process until partially smoothed, about 1 1/2 minutes.
5. Cut the cream cheese into 9 or 10 chunks. One at a time, add the chunks through the feed tube. Process after each addition. Process until smooth—an additional 1 1/2–2 minutes.
6. Carefully spoon the mixture over the ground pecans.
7. Bake in the center of the preheated oven for 15 minutes.
8. Lower the oven temperature to 325 degrees and bake for an additional 50 to 60 minutes or until the cheesecake edges have begun to brown and the center is puffed and seems set when the surface is lightly tapped.
9. Remove to a rack and cool for 20 minutes. Refrigerate at least 6 hours or overnight until cooled. When cooled, cover with plastic wrap.
10. If desired, top with cut fruit.

Preparation Time:
10 minutes

Serves 8

Serving Size:
2 Tbsp

Dessert Sauce for Fruit

For an easy and elegant sauce that tastes wonderful on strawberries or mixed fruit, try this sweetened mixture of sour cream and ricotta cheese. The recipe is easy to double if you want to serve it at a party. Because the sauce contains ricotta cheese, be sure to process it for at least a minute and a half so the texture will be smooth.

1 cup reduced-fat sour cream

1/4 cup part-skim ricotta cheese

3 Tbsp Splenda

1/2 tsp vanilla extract

1. In a food processor bowl, combine the sour cream, ricotta, Splenda, and vanilla.
2. Process until smooth, at least 1 1/2 minutes, stopping once and scraping down the sides of the container with a rubber spatula. Transfer to a small bowl and refrigerate, or serve at once on fruit.

Exchanges

1 Fat

Calories 48

Total Fat 3 g

Saturated Fat 2 g

Calories from Fat 28

Cholesterol 12 mg

Sodium 30 mg

Carbohydrate 3 g

Dietary Fiber 0 g

Sugars 2 g

Protein 3 g

Greek-Style Quiche

Preparation Time: 15 minutes without crust

Serves 9

Serving Size: 1/9 quiche

This quiche is good with or without a crust. You can use the pastry crust on p. 206, or simply pour the quiche right into the plate and bake it.

1 Easy Pastry Crust (see recipe, p. 206)
1 1/2 cups frozen cut-leaf spinach
1 cup liquid egg substitute
3/4 cup reduced-fat ricotta cheese
2 Tbsp white flour
1 1/4 cups shredded part-skim mozzarella cheese
1 cup crumbled feta cheese
1 Tbsp olive oil
1 1/2 tsp dried dill weed
1 tsp minced garlic

1. Prepare the pastry crust at least 20 minutes before needed.
2. Preheat the oven to 350 degrees. For a crustless quiche, spray a 9-inch pie plate with nonstick spray and set aside.
3. Place the spinach in a small microwave-safe bowl, cover with wax paper, and microwave on 30 percent power for 4 or 5 minutes, or until the spinach is thawed. Press the excess water from the spinach.
4. In a large bowl, stir together the egg substitute, ricotta, and flour. Stir in the mozzarella, feta, olive oil, dill, and garlic. Stir in the spinach.
5. Transfer to the pie plate. Bake for 35 to 40 minutes until set, browned around the edges, and firm in the middle.

Exchanges (with crust)
1 Starch
2 Lean Meat
1 1/2 Fat

Calories 250
Total Fat 14 g
Saturated Fat 5 g
Calories from Fat 130
Cholesterol 28 mg
Sodium 394 mg
Carbohydrate 16 g
Dietary Fiber 2 g
Sugars 3 g
Protein 15 g

Exchanges (without crust)
2 Lean Meat
1/2 Carbohydrate

Calories 136
Total Fat 7 g
Saturated Fat 4 g
Calories from Fat 67
Cholesterol 28 mg
Sodium 326 mg
Carbohydrate 6 g
Dietary Fiber 1 g
Sugars 2 g
Protein 13 g

Preparation Time: 12 minutes

Serves 30

Serving Size: 1 piece

Exchanges

1 Fat

Calories 38

Total Fat 3 g

Saturated Fat 0 g

Calories from Fat 26

Cholesterol 0 mg

Sodium 3 mg

Carbohydrate 2 g

Dietary Fiber 1 g

Sugars 1 g

Protein 1 g

Marzipan Candy

One of my favorite candies is marzipan. So I was excited to devise this easy, delicious, and sugar-free method of making it.

1 6-oz package blanched, slivered almonds

1 cup Splenda

2 Tbsp liquid egg substitute

2 tsp almond extract

1 tsp lemon juice

1. In food processor, process the almonds until very finely ground. Turn off the machine and add the Splenda, egg substitute, almond extract, and lemon juice. Process until the mixture forms a ball, or is well combined.
2. Transfer to a 1-quart or similar microwave-safe shallow casserole or plastic container. Press the marzipan into place. Cover with wax paper and microwave about 4 minutes at 30 percent power, until firm but not dry. Cool. With a sharp knife, cut into squares.
3. Store tightly covered in the refrigerator. Marzipan will keep for up to 10 days.

Marzipan Crust

I use this wonderful crust for both my fruit tart and my cranberry-orange tart.

1 6-oz package blanched, slivered almonds

1/4 cup liquid egg substitute

1/3 cup Splenda

2 Tbsp warm water

1 tsp almond extract

1. In a food processor, process the almonds until they are very finely ground.
2. Turn off the machine and add the egg substitute, Splenda, water, and almond extract. Process until well combined.
3. Transfer to a 9- or 10-inch microwave-safe dinner plate. Pat and shape into a circle with a slight raised area at the edge. Cover with wax paper and microwave on high power about 2 minutes or until the crust is somewhat firm. If the crust has risen from center of plate, press it back into place.
4. Continue to microwave, covered with wax paper, in 30-second increments, until the crust is almost dry in the center, about 1 to 2 more minutes. Set the plate on a wire rack to cool slightly.

Preparation Time: 10 minutes

Serves 8

Serving Size: 1/8 crust

Exchanges

2 Fat

Calories 135

Total Fat 11 g

Saturated Fat 0 g

Calories from Fat 99

Cholesterol 0 mg

Sodium 17 mg

Carbohydrate 6 g

Dietary Fiber 3 g

Sugars 2 g

Protein 4

Preparation Time: 20 minutes

Serves 8

Serving Size: 1/8 pie

Exchanges

1 Starch

1 1/2 Fat

Calories 128

Total Fat 8 g

Saturated Fat 1 g

Calories from Fat 72

Cholesterol 0 mg

Sodium 76 mg

Carbohydrate 11 g

Dietary Fiber 1 g

Sugars 2 g

Protein 3 g

Easy Pastry Crust

I've always considered traditional pie crust one of the least nutritious foods you could eat, since it's sky-high in both fat and carb. Here's one that's better for you. There's relatively little fat and some protein from the soy flour, which is available at health-food stores. Another plus is that the crust is relatively thin, especially when made in a deep-dish pie plate. This recipe makes crust for a 9-inch or 9-inch deep-dish pie.

If you hate rolling out pie crust the way I do, you'll find this one easy to make, because you mix it right in the pie plate and then press it into place. When I make the crust, I distribute most of the mixture over the bottom and sides of the plate, then press the sides into place first, using my thumb to hold the upper edge in place as I work. When the sides are in place, I smooth out the bottom of the crust. Finally, I press the crust down around the edges of the plate with a fork to make an attractive edge.

3/4 cup white flour

1/2 cup soy flour

1/4 tsp salt

1/4 cup canola oil

2 Tbsp plus 2 tsp fat-free milk (or a little more if necessary)

1. In a 9-inch pie plate or deep-dish pie plate, carefully stir together the flours and salt with a fork.
2. In a 1-cup measure, beat together the oil and milk with a fork, until the milk is completely incorporated.
3. Gradually add the oil mixture to the flours, stirring with a spoon as you pour it in. Use your fingers to finish working the liquid into the dry ingredients. If the mixture will not hold together, add a few more drops of milk to make it workable. But do not over-moisten the pastry.
4. When the ingredients are well blended, press the mixture into place in the pie plate with your fingers, working it out evenly over the sides and bottom and over the top edge. Crimp the edge with the tines of a fork.
5. Lightly cover with plastic wrap and allow to rest at room temperature 10 to 20 minutes while you prepare the filling ingredients.
6. Follow recipe directions for specific pie.

Preparation Time:
12 minutes

Serves 7

Serving Size:
1 cup

Mulled "Cider"

I've always loved the taste of hot mulled cider. This hot winter drink tastes a lot like traditional mulled cider, but has fewer calories. It's easy to double the recipe if you want to serve a large pot of this flavorful hot punch.

6 cups hot decaffeinated or caffeinated tea
1 cup orange juice
2 Tbsp lemon juice
3/4 cup Splenda, or to taste
1/2 tsp vanilla
1/4 tsp orange extract
1 cinnamon stick
6 whole cloves

1. Combine all the ingredients in a large saucepan. Bring to a simmer. Simmer for 20 minutes to allow the spices to permeate the liquid.
2. Ladle into mugs. Leftovers will keep in the refrigerator 2 to 3 days. Rewarm in the microwave.

Exchanges

1/2 Carbohydrate

Calories 30
Total Fat 0 g
Saturated Fat 0 g
Calories from Fat 1
Cholesterol 0 mg
Sodium 7 mg
Carbohydrate 7 g
Dietary Fiber 0 g
Sugars 6 g
Protein 0 g

Peanut Butter and Marmalade Sandwich

Preparation Time: 5 minutes

Serves 1

Serving Size: 1 open-faced sandwich

This is one of my favorite snack recipes, because it has the taste of peanut butter and marmalade without any extra sugar.

2 Tbsp natural peanut butter, at room temperature

1 tsp Splenda, or to taste

1/8 tsp orange extract, or to taste

1 small slice whole-wheat bread

1. In a small bowl, blend the peanut butter, Splenda, and orange extract together with a fork.
2. Spread on whole-wheat bread.

Exchanges

1 Starch

2 High-Fat Meat

Calories 262

Total Fat 17 g

Saturated Fat 2 g

Calories from Fat 155

Cholesterol 0 mg

Sodium 268 mg

Carbohydrate 19 g

Dietary Fiber 4 g

Sugars 4 g

Protein 11 g

Preparation Time: 5 minutes

Serves 1

Serving Size: 1 cup

Curried Peanut Soup

Quick, easy, and tangy, this soup is great for a cold winter day. I prefer to make it with peanut butter that hasn't been refrigerated. If you have only refrigerated peanut butter, you will need to bring it to room temperature in the microwave before making the soup.

2 Tbsp fat-free sour cream

1 Tbsp natural peanut butter, at room temperature

1/2 tsp mild curry powder, or to taste

1 cup reduced-sodium chicken broth

1. In a small bowl, whisk together the sour cream, peanut butter, and curry powder until smooth.
2. Gradually whisk in the chicken broth until well combined.
3. Microwave 1 minute.
4. Pour into a mug.

Exchanges

1 High-Fat Meat

1/2 Carbohydrate

Calories 138

Total Fat 8 g

Saturated Fat 1 g

Calories from Fat 73

Cholesterol 2 mg

Sodium 595 mg

Carbohydrate 9 g

Dietary Fiber 1 g

Sugars 4 g

Protein 7 g

Pecan Pie Crust

This richly-flavored crust makes a nice change from a graham cracker crust.

Crust for 9-inch pie

1 1/4 cups very finely ground pecans

2 Tbsp Splenda

2 Tbsp melted reduced-fat margarine or butter

Crust for 9-inch deep-dish pie

2 cups very finely ground pecans

3 Tbsp plus 1 tsp Splenda

3 Tbsp plus 1 tsp melted reduced-fat margarine or butter

1. Preheat the oven to 400 degrees.
2. In a small bowl, mix together the pecans and Splenda. Stir in the butter. Moisten your fingers with water and press the mixture firmly against the bottom and sides of the pie plate. Quickly press a base of crust into the flat portion of the plate. Then work some of the mixture up the sides of the plate. Finally, return to the middle, and smooth out the crust into a thin layer. If the crust sticks to your fingers, moisten them again. If the crust is for an unbaked pie filling, bake the crust until it is lightly browned, about 6 to 8 minutes.

Preparation Time: 20 minutes

Serves 1

Serving Size: 1/8 crust (regular); 1/9 crust (deep-dish)

Exchanges (regular pie)

2 1/2 Fat

Calories 118
Total Fat 12 g
Saturated Fat 1 g
Calories from Fat 110
Cholesterol 0 mg
Sodium 19 mg
Carbohydrate 2 g
Dietary Fiber 1 g
Sugars 1 g
Protein 1 g

Exchanges (deep-dish pie)

3 1/2 Fat

Calories 168
Total Fat 18 g
Saturated Fat 2 g
Calories from Fat 158
Cholesterol 0 mg
Sodium 28 mg
Carbohydrate 3 g
Dietary Fiber 2 g
Sugars 1 g
Protein 2 g

Preparation Time: 10 minutes

Serves 12

Serving Size: 6 nut halves

Spiced Pecans

Be careful; these sweetened pecan halves are addictive. The recipe calls for butter, but only a very small amount per serving is used. And some of the fat is blotted away when the nuts are spread on a paper towel after cooking.

1 1/2 Tbsp butter

1 tsp pumpkin pie spice

2 cups pecan halves

1/2 Tbsp sugar-free pancake syrup

1/2 tsp vanilla extract

1. Set out a dinner plate covered with a paper towel.
2. In a large skillet, melt the butter over medium heat. Stir in the pumpkin pie spice. Stir in the pecans and cook, stirring, over medium to medium-high heat for 5 minutes, until nuts are sautéed and the flavors are blended.
3. Add the syrup and vanilla and continue to cook, stirring for an additional 1 to 1 1/2 minutes.
4. Transfer the nuts to the plate, spreading them out. Allow to cool. Store in a tightly closed container in the refrigerator. Nuts will keep for several weeks.

Exchanges

3 Fat

Calories 142

Total Fat 15 g

Saturated Fat 2 g

Calories from Fat 133

Cholesterol 4 mg

Sodium 15 mg

Carbohydrate 3 g

Dietary Fiber 2 g

Sugars 1 g

Protein 2 g

Salmon Spread

You can enjoy this tasty spread as either an appetizer or a snack.

1 6-oz can boneless, skinless salmon, drained

3 oz reduced-fat cream cheese, cut into 3 or 4 pieces

1 tsp lemon juice

1 tsp instant minced onion

1/4 tsp dried dill weed

1 tsp prepared white horseradish

1/8 tsp salt, or to taste

2 to 3 drops hot pepper sauce

3 Tbsp chopped pecans

1/4 cup finely chopped celery

1. In a food processor container, combine the salmon, cream cheese, lemon juice, onion, dill, horseradish, salt, and hot pepper sauce. Process until almost completely smooth. Stir in the pecans and celery.
2. Transfer to a small serving bowl. Serve with crackers or celery sticks. Serve at once or cover and refrigerate. Spread will keep in the refrigerator for 4 to 5 days.

Preparation Time: 15 minutes

Serves 24

Serving Size: 2 tsp (as an appetizer)

Serves 8

Serving Size: 2 Tbsp (as a snack)

Exchanges (appetizer)
1/2 Fat

Calories 26
Total Fat 2 g
Saturated Fat 1 g
Calories from Fat 17
Cholesterol 7 mg
Sodium 69 mg
Carbohydrate 0 g
Dietary Fiber 0 g
Sugars 0 g
Protein 2 g

Exchanges (snack)
1 Lean Meat
1/2 Fat

Calories 78
Total Fat 51 g
Saturated Fat 2 g
Calories from Fat 51
Cholesterol 20 mg
Sodium 208 mg
Carbohydrate 1 g
Dietary Fiber 0 g
Sugars 1 g
Protein 6 g

Summer Cheesecake

Preparation Time: 20 minutes

Serves 9

Serving Size: 1/9 pie

Light summer cheesecake is one of my old favorite desserts. This version has a wonderful flavor, even though the sugar and much of the fat have been eliminated. One of the ingredients is evaporated fat-free milk. When chilled very cold, it can be whipped just like cream. If you want to be sure the milk is cold enough, chill it until ice crystals begin to form around the edges. By the way, be sure to lightly whip the milk. If you whip it too much, you will have more filling than will fit into the pie shell. If you have extra filling, simply pour any leftovers into a small glass bowl, and refrigerate it separately.

1 9-inch deep-dish Pecan Pie Crust (see recipe, p. 211)

1 12-oz can evaporated fat-free milk, divided

2 packets unflavored gelatin

1 cup boiling water

1/4 cup lemon juice

1 8-oz package reduced-fat cream cheese, cut into 3 or 4 pieces

1 cup Splenda

1 Tbsp vanilla

Exchanges

4 1/2 Fat

1 Carbohydrate

Calories 281

Total Fat 23 g

Saturated Fat 5 g

Calories from Fat 206

Cholesterol 18 mg

Sodium 192 mg

Carbohydrate 12 g

Dietary Fiber 2 g

Sugars 9 g

Protein 9 g

1. Make deep-dish Pecan Pie Crust. Set aside.
2. Pour 1/4 cup of the milk into a food processor bowl and set aside. Pour the remaining milk into a mixing bowl (preferably metal) and put it into the freezer.
3. Combine the gelatin and boiling water in a measuring cup. Stir until the gelatin is dissolved, about 1 or 2 minutes. Add the lemon juice. Reserve.
4. To the food processor bowl, add the cream cheese, Splenda, and vanilla. Process until smooth, about 2 minutes. Pour in the gelatin mixture through the feed tube. Process until well combined.
5. When the remaining evaporated milk is very cold, beat on high speed with an electric mixer until lightly whipped, about a minute and a half. Reduce the speed to medium. With mixer running, beat in the cream cheese mixture.
6. Pour the mixture into the prepared pie crust. Refrigerate until set, about 2 hours. Cover. Cheesecake will keep in the refrigerator for 3 to 4 days.

Sweet Potato Pie

Preparation Time: 25 minutes

Serves 9

Serving Size: 1/9 pie or custard

Exchanges (with crust)

1 1/2 Fat

2 Carbohydrate

Calories 209

Total Fat 7 g

Saturated Fat 1 g

Calories from Fat 65

Cholesterol 0 mg

Sodium 151 mg

Carbohydrate 28 g

Dietary Fiber 2 g

Sugars 12 g

Protein 8 g

Exchanges (without crust)

1 Carbohydrate

Calories 95

Total Fat 0 g

Saturated Fat 0 g

Calories from Fat 2

Cholesterol 0 mg

Sodium 84 mg

Carbohydrate 18 g

Dietary Fiber 1 g

Sugars 11 g

Protein 5 g

This recipe is a little more work than some. But it's worth it, because sweet potatoes are so good for you and because the pie tastes so delicious. I use fresh sweet potatoes and microwave them while I'm preparing the other ingredients. Two cups is about 2 large sweet potatoes.

To make this recipe easier, you can turn it into a custard by leaving off the crust. For both the custard and the pie, I use a 9-inch deep-dish pie plate.

1 Easy Pastry Crust (see recipe, p. 206)

1/2 cup liquid egg substitute

1 12-oz can evaporated fat-free milk

1 tsp vanilla extract

2 cups cooked, mashed sweet potato

2/3 cup Splenda

2 tsp pumpkin pie spice

1/2 tsp ground ginger

1. If making a pie, prepare the pastry crust at least 20 minutes before needed. If making a custard, spray the pie plate with nonstick spray and set aside. Preheat the oven to 350 degrees.
2. In a 2-cup measure or similar small bowl, combine the egg substitute, milk, and vanilla. Set aside.
3. Place the sweet potatoes in a mixer bowl and beat slightly at low speed to smooth. Add the Splenda, pumpkin pie spice, ginger, and about 1/2 cup of the milk mixture, continuing to beat at medium speed. When incorporated, slowly beat in the remaining milk mixture, stopping and scraping down the sides and bottom of the bowl as necessary, beating about 4 or 5 minutes until the mixture is smooth.
4. Pour the filling into the pie plate and bake in the center of the oven for 42 to 45 minutes or until set and browned around the edges. A toothpick inserted in the center should come out clean.

Preparation Time: 5 minutes

Serves 2

Serving Size: 1/2 cup

Quick Sweet Potato Snacks

Try this easy and very tasty way to enjoy a sweet potato. Microwave cooking makes preparation a snap.

1 medium sweet potato

1 tsp Splenda

1 tsp olive oil

1/2 tsp orange extract

1/4 tsp pumpkin pie spice

2 Tbsp chopped pecans or walnuts

1. Lay the sweet potato on a plate. Pierce the potato in several places with a knife or a fork. Microwave on high power about 7 minutes or until cooked through.
2. Cut the sweet potato in half. Scoop out the flesh onto a medium-sized plate. Mash with a fork.
3. Mash in the Splenda, oil, orange extract, and pumpkin pie spice. Stir in the nuts. Leftovers can be covered, refrigerated, and reheated in the microwave.

Exchanges

1 Starch

1 1/2 Fat

Calories 133

Total Fat 8 g

Saturated Fat 1 g

Calories from Fat 68

Cholesterol 0 mg

Sodium 6 mg

Carbohydrate 15 g

Dietary Fiber 2 g

Sugars 7 g

Protein 2 g

Teriyaki Chicken Bites

These tasty chicken bites are great party food. You can make them in the broiler, but they cook much more quickly in a George Foreman grill.

3 Tbsp lite soy sauce

2 Tbsp peanut oil

1 tsp rice vinegar or white vinegar

1 tsp Splenda

1/2 tsp ground ginger

1 tsp minced garlic

1 lb boneless, skinless chicken breast

1. In a large bowl or ceramic casserole, mix together the soy sauce, oil, vinegar, Splenda, ginger, and garlic.
2. With a sharp knife, cut the chicken into bite-sized pieces.
3. Put the chicken into the bowl with the marinade. Stir to coat. Cover and refrigerate 2 to 3 hours or up to 12 hours, stirring occasionally.
4. If broiling, transfer the chicken and marinade to a 9 1/2 × 13-inch baking pan. Broil about 4 inches from the heat, turning chicken and basting occasionally with the sauce, for 17 to 20 minutes until the chicken pieces are cooked through and begin to brown. If using a George Foreman grill, grill about 5 to 6 minutes. Serve warm with toothpicks. Chicken can be cooked ahead and reheated in the broiler or microwave.

Preparation Time: 15 minutes

Serves 6

Serving Size: 4 pieces

Exchanges

2 Lean Meat

Calories 119

Total Fat 5 g

Saturated Fat 1 g

Calories from Fat 44

Cholesterol 46 mg

Sodium 242 mg

Carbohydrate 1 g

Dietary Fiber 0 g

Sugars 1 g

Protein 17 g

Preparation Time: 8 minutes

Serves 2

Serving Size: scant 1 cup

Exchanges

1 High-Fat Meat

1/2 Carbohydrate

Calories 135

Total Fat 9 g

Saturated Fat 1 g

Calories from Fat 77

Cholesterol 2 mg

Sodium 343 mg

Carbohydrate 9 g

Dietary Fiber 2 g

Sugars 6 g

Protein 6 g

Tomato Soup with a Difference

This recipe may look unusual, but the peanut butter added to this tomato soup gives it a very pleasing flavor. I use a large saucepan to give myself ample room for whisking.

2 Tbsp natural peanut butter, at room temperature

1 cup reduced-sodium or regular chicken broth

1/2 cup low-sodium or regular tomato sauce

1/4 cup reduced-fat (2%) milk

Dash onion powder

2 to 3 drops hot pepper sauce

1. Place the peanut butter in a large saucepan. Warm over medium-low heat. Slowly whisk in 1/3 of the chicken broth at a time, whisking well after each addition, until blended. If the peanut butter will not combine, transfer to a blender. Blend on high speed about 1 minute or until smooth before returning the mixture to the pan.
2. Add the tomato sauce, milk, onion powder, and hot pepper sauce. Heat until warmed.
3. Pour into two mugs and serve.

Mexican Tuna Dip

Preparation Time:
10 minutes

Serves 10

Serving Size:
2 Tbsp

In La Paz, Mexico, while you sit in a restaurant and contemplate the sea and palm trees, you can enjoy an interesting variation on the standard chips and dip appetizer. Instead of salsa, the waiter is likely to set out a creamy dip that's enlivened with canned tuna. Here's my version. At home, I serve this dip with celery sticks, broccoli, and cauliflower as well as fat-free baked corn chips.

1/2 cup reduced-fat mayonnaise

1/4 cup reduced-fat sour cream

3 Tbsp mild or medium salsa

2 tsp Splenda

2 tsp cider vinegar

1 6-oz can albacore tuna, drained and flaked

1. Mix together the mayonnaise, sour cream, and salsa. Stir in the Splenda and vinegar. Stir in the tuna. Serve at once or refrigerate. Dip will keep in the refrigerator for 2 to 3 days.
2. Serve with fat-free tortilla chips or vegetables. For a larger snack portion, spread 3 Tbsp on a piece of whole-wheat bread.

Exchanges

1 Very Lean Meat

1 Fat

Calories 66

Total Fat 5 g

Saturated Fat 1 g

Calories from Fat 42

Cholesterol 10 mg

Sodium 164 mg

Carbohydrate 2 g

Dietary Fiber 0 g

Sugars 0 g

Protein 4 g

Index

ALPHABETICAL LIST OF RECIPES

SUBJECT INDEX

About the American Diabetes Association

The American Diabetes Association is the nation's leading voluntary health organization supporting diabetes research, information, and advocacy. Its mission is to prevent and cure diabetes and to improve the lives of all people affected by diabetes. The American Diabetes Association is the leading publisher of comprehensive diabetes information. Its huge library of practical and authoritative books for people with diabetes covers every aspect of self-care—cooking and nutrition, fitness, weight control, medications, complications, emotional issues, and general self-care.

To order American Diabetes Association books: Call 1-800-232-6733.
Or log on to http://store.diabetes.org

To join the American Diabetes Association: Call 1-800-806-7801.
www.diabetes.org/membership

For more information about diabetes or ADA programs and services:
Call 1-800-342-2383. E-mail: Customerservice@diabetes.org or log on to www.diabetes.org

To locate an ADA/NCQA Recognized Provider of quality diabetes care in your area: www.ncqa.org/dprp/

To find an ADA Recognized Education Program in your area:
Call 1-888-232-0822. www.diabetes.org/recognition/education.asp

To join the fight to increase funding for diabetes research, end discrimination, and improve insurance coverage: Call 1-800-342-2383.
www.diabetes.org/advocacy

To find out how you can get involved with the programs in your community: Call 1-800-342-2383. See below for program Web addresses.

- *American Diabetes Month:* Educational activities aimed at those diagnosed with diabetes—month of November. www.diabetes.org/ADM
- *American Diabetes Alert:* Annual public awareness campaign to find the undiagnosed—held the fourth Tuesday in March. www.diabetes.org/alert
- *The Diabetes Assistance & Resources Program (DAR):* diabetes awareness program targeted to the Latino community. www.diabetes.org/DAR
- *African American Program:* diabetes awareness program targeted to the African American community. www.diabetes.org/africanamerican
- *Awakening the Spirit: Pathways to Diabetes Prevention & Control:* diabetes awareness program targeted to the Native American community. www.diabetes.org/awakening

To find out about an important research project regarding type 2 diabetes:
www.diabetes.org/ada/research.asp

To obtain information on making a planned gift or charitable bequest:
Call 1-888-700-7029. www.diabetes.org/ada/plan.asp

To make a donation or memorial contribution: Call 1-800-342-2383.
www.diabetes.org/ada/cont.asp